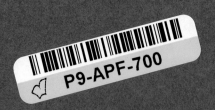

UNSHIELDED:
THE HUMAN COST OF THE DALKON SHIELD

Promoted as the 'Cadillac of contraception,' the Dalkon Shield intrauterine device was used by four million women worldwide between 1970
and 1974. However, physicians and women were not warned of its dangers. Many users suffered from pelvic inflammatory disease, septic
abortions, infertility, and other physical problems as a result of the
Dalkon Shield's faulty design. To date, 300,000 women have filed a
class action suit against the manufacturer, A.H. Robins, for causing
bodily harm, and 200,000 women have received monetary compensation
from the Dalkon Shield Claimants Trust.

While there have been other accounts of the legal proceedings and
medical controversies, this is the first book that focuses on the human
costs of the Dalkon Shield in the aftermath of the class action suit. Mary
Hawkins reveals that many women did not have adequate legal representation. Medical records had been destroyed and women were treated
dismissively by the medical committee responsible for compensation.
Some lawyers seized on the Dalkon Shield claims as a get-rich-quick
scheme. As a result, many women lost faith in the Canadian and American medical and legal systems. Finally, Hawkins addresses the emotional injuries sustained by the women and by their partners. She brings
together stories from survivors as well as critical analysis of the media
and of the medical and legal systems at the root of the fiasco.

Unshielded: The Human Cost of the Dalkon Shield provides a comprehensive overview of the manufacturing and marketing of the IUD,
and its trail of destruction. It brings to life a story that has been obscured
by legal and medical bureaucracy and presents an important lesson
about the impact of misinformation on the public.

MARY F. HAWKINS teaches at the postsecondary level and is a communi-
cations consultant and researcher/writer in Ottawa.

MARY F. HAWKINS

Unshielded:
The Human Cost of the
Dalkon Shield

UNIVERSITY OF TORONTO PRESS
Toronto Buffalo London

© University of Toronto Press Incorporated 1997
Toronto Buffalo London
Printed in Canada

ISBN 0-8020-0876-3 (cloth)
ISBN 0-8020-7861-3 (paper)

Printed on acid-free paper

Canadian Cataloguing in Publication Data

Hawkins, Mary F. (Mary Florence), 1953–
    Unshielded: the human cost of the Dalkon Shield

    Includes bibliographical references and index.
    ISBN 0-8020-0876-3 (bound) ISBN 0-8020-7861-3 (pbk.)

    1. A.H. Robins Company.   2. Dalkon Shield (Intrauterine
    contraceptive).   3. Intrauterine contraceptives –
    Complications.   4. Intrauterine contraceptives industry –
    United States.   I. Title.

    HD9995.C64A235 1997   338.7'616139435   C97-931342-2

University of Toronto Press acknowledges the financial assistance to its
publishing program of the Canada Council and the Ontario Arts Council.

For the survivors of the Dalkon Shield
May a healing spirit embrace you.

Contents

Preface

When I began to research the story of the Dalkon Shield I had no concept of the vastness of the information and the complex relationships among the various players and events. I had no idea of the depth and breadth of pain felt by so many of the women who were affected. I did not know the interrelationships among the various people involved, nor did I realize the social, economic, and political ramifications of these relationships. Most of all, I did not know of the vast numbers of women who were literally and figuratively isolated from others with the same experience.

The realization that there were hundreds of thousands of women worldwide from diverse cultures, but with common experiences, was astounding. Receiving letters from women living in isolated rural areas of Canada brought tears to my eyes. It was the first time many of these women had had an opportunity to share their experiences with another person. Although these women were separated from one another, they represented a female collective – a sisterhood – in pursuit of acknowledgment of and compensation for personal injury. The image of hundreds of thousands of women around the globe taking a stand against a large American corporation sent a powerful message not only to corporate America but also to women at large. It was exhilarating to see – despite resistance from political and economic factions in industry and government – that these women together were able to manoeuvre a company such as A.H. Robins Pharmaceutical Co. into bankruptcy.

The background research on the Dalkon Shield and interviews with more than 100 Canadians and Americans have provided a cross-section of information for this book. The interviews provide a personal dimension to a story that reveals the tragic human costs of the Dalkon Shield. Very few people when personally contacted declined to be interviewed, although some wished to remain anonymous.

The writing of *Unshielded* was an intriguing and, at times, an intense experience. To learn that so many people suffered so much because of senseless action and inaction by corporate entities was mind-boggling and, at the same time, gut-wrenching. There certainly were times when I asked myself and friends why I was delving into such a complex story. Ultimately I was able to do it primarily because of my inner conviction that the public must know about certain injustices. They must also know, through the example of others, that the fight for justice can succeed if people take collective action. It is crucial that the lessons learned and not learned from tragedies such as that of the Dalkon Shield fiasco are recognized by consumers, business, government, and the health-care industry. We have choices about how to treat our bodies. The key to making wise choices is developing a strong information base about what will benefit our well-being in both the short and the long term.

Acknowledgments

My everlasting appreciation goes to the women who contributed their Dalkon Shield stories as background information for this book. They will always be remembered for their courage. Thank you also to Gerry for sharing the story of his pain and healing over the loss of his son. His contribution will no doubt assist other men who have not yet been able to speak out about their own experiences.

Thank you to Laura Jones, Doris R. Hawkins, and Dr Nedra Lander for their editorial comments and patience. Their feedback and support has been invaluable. Laura Jones opened her home to me so that I could meet and interview the Dalkon Shield Action Canada (DSAC) activist members who fought so hard for their convictions. The contributions of all of the DSAC group are deeply appreciated. Much gratitude to my mother, Doris Hawkins, who patiently listened while I rambled on about the details of the book and for her keen proofreading skills. My close friend and mentor Nedra Lander's candid comments, moral support, and enthusiasm for this project often provided a light at the end of the tunnel.

Thank you to Giles Daigle for his enthusiasm and legal advice about the intricacies of writing a book. My appreciation is extended to the many Dalkon Shield lawyers who provided insight into the legal aspects of the litigation, as well as to the physicians and health educators who had the courage to speak out.

Marilyn Grant and Claudia Kutchukian deserve special thanks for providing their invaluable editorial expertise to the overall manuscript. I also want to thank research assistants Melanie Scott and Elizabeth Lander. My appreciation to Kathy Sperberg for catalogue assistance. Thank you to Jennifer P. for listening and for her wonderful intuition, as well as to other friends and acquaintances who have stood by me in the process of bringing this manuscript together. Thank you to my thirteen-year-old godson, Jonathan Line, for his inspirational words 'You can do it.' My appreciation to Dr Susan Sollars for being such a wonderful family physician. Thank you to Virgil Duff, Executive Managing Editor, University of Toronto Press for his faith in this project from beginning to end. My gratitude to all of the University of Toronto Press staff for their efforts in packaging the final book. My appreciation to the Ontario Arts Council, Writers Reserve Program, for financial assistance.

Finally, I would like to express my gratitude to the following people for their individual and collective comments: Dr Arthur Leader, MD; Dr Norman Barwin, MD; Dr Paul Claman, MD; Dr Marion Powell, MD; Dr Jeffrey Turnbull, MD; Dr Michael Moreton, MD; Dr Pierre Tremblay, MD; Dr Sydney Kronick, MD; Dr W.L. Sim, MD; Dr Brian Ivey, MD; Dr Carolyn De Marco, MD; Dr Dorothy Shaw, MD; Dr Susan Roche, MD; Dr Pierre Blais, PhD; Dr Pat Gervaize, PhD; Dr William Freeland, MD, Chief, Device Evaluation Division, Health Canada; Ann Malo, MA; Richard Tobin, Director, Medical Devices Bureau, Health Canada; Barb Dimambro, MSW; Miles Lord, LLB; Robert Montague, LLB; Carey Linde, LLB; Christopher Kay, LLB; Gaetan Duschene, LLB; Michael Leff, LLB; Mike Pretl, LLB; John Baker, LLB; and Sybil Shainwald, LLB. Thank you also to Joel Duff; Michael McBane, Canadian Health Coalition; and activists Belita Cowan (founder of the National Women's Health Network), Susan Russell (Canadian Federation of Women), Dr Karen Hicks, PhD, (founder of the Dalkon Shield Information Network (DSIN)), Linda Hightower, (Dalkon Shield Victims), Dr Kathy Kaby Anselmi, PhD, Dolores Vader, Cathy Cameron, and Ivy Tremaine; Madelaine Bosco of the Women's Health Clinic, Manitoba, Canada; Dr Madeline Weld, PhD, Global Concerns; Bonnie Johnson, Planned Parenthood Federation of Canada; Jill Weiss, Canadian PID Society; Marcena Croy, Planned Parenthood Federation, Vancouver, BC; Trish Maynard, Fertility Awareness Association of Canada; T. Polhill, RNA, Birth Control Victims Association of Canada; Farahana Rana, research support, and Heather Broughton, former editor of Canadian Nurses Association; Society of Obstetrics/Gynecology, Canada; and Karen Alcon, American Health Industry Manufacturers Association.

MARY F. HAWKINS

UNSHIELDED:
THE HUMAN COST OF THE DALKON SHIELD

Introduction

The story of the Dalkon Shield began in the late 1960s when a physician, Dr Hugh Davis, developed an intra-uterine device (IUD) that was said to provide a breakthrough in preventing pregnancy in women. With its design, the Dalkon Shield was promoted by its inventors and marketers as having a low expulsion and pregnancy rate. Despite promises and acclaim accompanying the release of the Dalkon Shield, its use devastated the lives of many women and their families.

Most women who were of child-bearing age in the early 1970s have heard of the Dalkon Shield. They either used it or know of someone who used it. Most of these women believed that the Dalkon Shield would offer them a safe and responsible means of birth control. For some of these women, however, the outcome was tragic. Some died; others incurred septic abortions, miscarriages, or chronic pelvic inflammatory disease (PID). Most of them lost the ability to have children.

Outraged, many Dalkon Shield users joined together in filing one of the largest lawsuits of its kind against the manufacturer of the Dalkon Shield, the American pharmaceutical company A.H. Robins. In doing so, they did not anticipate that they would wait more than ten years to receive any monetary compensation for their injuries. In many cases, the compensation finally received was minimal. To this day, women who have been left childless, in ill health, and with deep emotional wounds still have not received a public apology from the A.H. Robins company.

The main thrust of the marketing of the Dalkon Shield took place within the United States, but four million women worldwide used this

IUD. Their reasons for avoiding pregnancy were often based on financial constraints. Other women did not want to bear children out of
wedlock. Social mores of the 1960s and 1970s were such that many
young women and men had more than one sexual partner. Unfortunately, many of the women did not know that IUDs do not protect
their users from sexually transmitted diseases. The risk of sexually
transmitted disease and the properties of the IUD increased the
chances of pelvic inflammatory disease. In the case of the Dalkon
Shield, though, its properties alone are said to have been enough to
cause PID.

The litigation surrounding the Dalkon Shield continues to this day.
The removal of the Shield from the market was, for the most part, a
result of people speaking out. The women who filed suit against A.H.
Robins and the activists who protested the reorganization of the company's assets placed much of their emotional lives on hold in order to
see justice done. Some accepted minimal monetary compensation out of
naïvety about their legal rights. Others resisted the persuasive rhetoric of
the lawyers and the Dalkon Shield Claimants Trust officials to accept
low personal injury awards. Many women, determined to have their say
at a hearing or in court, waited and battled for years before receiving
compensation for their injuries. These women in some respects became
pioneers in their search for justice, establishing a foundation for future
and similar cases of personal injury.

Some lawyers battled alongside the activists. They vehemently
opposed A.H. Robins and the company's filing for bankruptcy under the
Chapter 11 bankruptcy code, which allowed Robins to reorganize its
assets. The company ended up selling its assets to American Home
Products for $3 billion, of which $2.45 billion was placed in a trust fund
for Dalkon Shield injury claims. Robins still walked away with $750
million. In this long and often bitter legal battle, lawyers played diverse
roles in a complex game of changing rules.

Along with lawyers and claimants, physicians had their own battles
to fight. Many had, in good faith, provided their patients with a presumably safe contraceptive. Letters from lawyers and patients demanding patients' medical files aroused fear and confusion. Physicians were
not used to this kind of demand on a large scale, especially those living in Canada. The alarm bells these demands set off resulted in physi-

cians' resisting handing over copies of patients' files to lawyers or to patients. The American Food and Drug Administration (FDA), the Canadian Health Protection Branch (HPB), medical insurance companies, Health maintenance organizations (HMOs) and medical protective associations received numerous letters and telephone calls from desperate physicians demanding advice on how to handle the requests from lawyers and patients. American and Canadian governmental bodies issued memos to physicians to stop using the Dalkon Shield. Despite the warning, physicians were not instructed to issue a recall on the Shield until some years later. During this period, a divisive attitude toward the Dalkon Shield developed in the medical community. Some held their own members accountable for using a device that appeared suspect.

The stories told by survivors of the Dalkon Shield draw an image of physicians making unnecessary moral judgments about their patients. Many physicians implied that these women incurred PID from promiscuous behaviour rather than from the Dalkon Shield. Feelings were hurt, resulting in conflicts between patients and physicians. As a result, the IUD as a contraceptive fell into disrepute among many in the patient community. Many within the medical community were disappointed, primarily because IUDs were a convenient and effective means of controlling unwanted pregnancies. Similarly, some pharmaceutical companies in the business of manufacturing IUDs reacted defensively by shifting their product lines to less controversial merchandise. The IUD, in essence, became a less profitable item to market.

The rise and fall of the Shield resulted in lessons both learned and ignored on the part of many of the players. This is evident in the context of the making and marketing of IUDs in general and the Dalkon Shield in particular; the litigation process; the healing of the survivors; and change or resistance within the medical community. Sadly, the lessons that were not learned from the Dalkon Shield experience seem to outweigh the lessons learned. Today, similar cases surround other medical devices or implants. One element of optimism nevertheless lies in the public's increased awareness of the health-care system. It also lies in an increased awareness among consumers that they can play a crucial role in deciding how they are medically treated.

We have learned that consumer education is a powerful force in enhancing the decision-making powers of the public. Evidently, we have also learned that we cannot depend on government or corporations alone to look after our needs or interests. Health-care regulation reforms are still in a state of flux. In order to trust again we must work together to avoid further tragedies within the health-care system.

1

Making and Marketing the Dalkon Shield

The Dalkon Shield was not the first intrauterine device to cause harm to women. Three such devices marketed during the 1970s carried the risk of introducing harmful bacteria into the uterus: the Dalkon Shield, the Majzlin Spring, and the Antigon-Fall (Tatum 1977; Perry and Dawson 1985). The Birnberg Bow and the Dalkon Shield had a reputation for high perforation rates (Tatum 1977). The Dalkon Shield, Majzlin Spring, and Antigon-Fall IUDs had tail strings that allegedly had a rapid wicking characteristic (Tatum 1977, 1975; Mintz 1985). One might compare this wicking phenomenon to an ignited dynamite stick. Once the bacteria moved its way into the uterus it spread like wildfire, inflaming the uterus. This resulted in severe pelvic inflammatory disease, which caused intense pain and, in some cases, death. Dr Howard Tatum (1977) recommended that such IUDs be surgically removed. For these reasons, each of these IUDs have, at one time or another, been discontinued.

The Dalkon Shield is the IUD that has gained the most notoriety. The litigation surrounding its damaging properties, the harm incurred by women who used the Shield, and the corporate deceit and lies revealed in the litigation process have all contributed to its infamous reputation (Mintz 1985; Perry and Dawson 1985; Sobol 1991; Hicks 1994). For some in the medical community, the Dalkon Shield remains an example of the drawbacks of most IUDs.

IUDs are small contraceptive devices that fit into the uterus. Some contain copper or synthetic progesterone, others are made only of white plastic, and most have one or more strings (Boston Women's Health

Book Collective 1992). 'No one is absolutely sure how the IUD works. The most widely accepted theory is that it causes an inflammation or chronic low-grade infection in the uterus. These cells may damage or destroy the sperm or egg and prevent them from joining' (Boston Women's Health Book Collective 1992, 295).

IUDs have been in use for over 2,000 years. Arabs and Turks used a form of an IUD on camels while on desert expeditions. According to a U.S. Food and Drug Administration (FDA) report, these devices included small stones that were inserted through a hollow tube into the uterus of the camel before crossing the desert to prevent pregnancy (Mintz 1985). Women have used IUDs since biblical times, according to the Old Testament. Materials women used over time included ebony, glass, gold, ivory, pewter, wood, wool, and diamond-studded platinum. Devices such as these also induced infection within the uterus. Despite this drawback, the scientific world persisted in attempting to perfect the design and materials of IUDs. Dr. Richard Richter is said to have discovered the principle of IUDs in 1909 (Davis 1972). An IUD made of silkworm gut created a flurry of interest in the early twentieth century within the medical community. This IUD, however, also tended to cause infection.

Another IUD, developed by Ernst Grafenberg in the early 1930s, caused a scare among the medical community. It was made of 'German silver,' which was a mixture of copper, silver, and zinc. It was also tailless, since Grafenberg felt that tail strings would encourage infection. In spite of this precaution, many women who wore the Grafenberg Ring experienced pain and infection. Grafenberg, like Hugh Davis in later years with the Dalkon Shield, predicted superior results with his invention; however, no one else was able to replicate his studies. As a result, the Grafenberg Ring was perceived as harmful by numerous physicians in the late 1930s. A standard textbook on contraception published in 1938 strongly recommended against its use (Perry and Dawson 1985). Because of such problems with IUDs, until 1958 they were considered to have little success and too many disadvantages as a contraceptive method.

The invention of the Japanese OTA Ring by Tenrei Takeo Ota in 1959 shifted perspectives on IUDs. It introduced two new design elements: a malleable inert plastic was used that was said to have a 'memory' of intended shape, along with a small-diameter inserter to place the IUD in the uterus. This 'memory' of intended shape meant that the plastic would likely mould to the shape of the uterus, and the inserter enabled the physician to insert the IUD with greater ease.

In order to establish evidence of the usefulness of the OTA IUD, 20,000 women were fitted with it. Although results from these experiments reported the OTA as being an excellent IUD, the scientists ignored failure rates by focusing primarily on the 'fine' material, plastic (Mintz 1985). The new materials allowed gynecologists and family physicians more ease in handling the device. They did not, as with other IUDs, have to open the cervix. 'With all earlier devices, including the Grafenberg ring, doctors had to insert a series of metal rods of increasing width in the opening of the woman's cervix to create a space wide enough for the IUD to pass through' (Perry and Dawson 1985, 14). In addition, antibiotics were available to counteract infection incurred from IUD insertion.

Evidence showed, however, that there was little comfort for the woman having the IUD inserted. It is commonly reported in many medical journals that severe cramping and, in some cases, excessive bleeding are frequent responses to the IUD. Nevertheless, excessive bleeding and cramping were the least of the problems for the women.

Around the mid-1800s scientists used slave women to test a newly developed IUD (Hicks 1994). Frequently, these women incurred severe infection and died as a result of the poor design of the IUD and the primitive medical procedures employed. According to Diane Scully, J. Marion Sims, an Alabama physician who has been called the father of gynecology, perfected gynecological surgery in the early 1850s. His subjects were slave women, 'a readily available source of material for experimentation. Without anesthesia, and with their owners' permission, he performed repeated surgical experiments on them. He was later praised as the "evangelist of healing to women"' (Hicks 1994, 18).

Dr Hugh Davis's subjects in the late 1960s included poor, mostly African-American, women from Baltimore's inner city (Hicks 1994; Mintz 1985). These women agreed to use the IUD in good faith, as did many women. One such woman believed Davis when he told her that her pain was all in her head. Mary Stone stated: 'He pointed to my head and said, "That's where your pain is!" In August 1975, I finally insisted on having it out. He was furious. He tore it out of me and threw it in the trash can' (Egan 1988 quoted in Hicks 1994). Prior to this incident, Davis had inserted three Dalkon Shields three separate times in this woman. On one of these occasions Davis could not locate the IUD; that is when he inserted the third one (Hicks 1994). Some women interviewed for this book also asserted that they had received similar treatment from some physicians when they asked to have the Dalkon Shield removed.

Many of these same women stated that information on the Dalkon Shield was inadequate. A simple brochure in the physician's office was often the only information available to them. Not only the adequacy but also the accuracy of information on the Shield was suspect, according to later scientific studies and written reports.

As a rule, adequate information produced from legitimate clinical studies is required from the U.S. Food and Drug Administration and the Canadian Health Protection Branch. These regulations suggest that scientists need to provide substantive data displaying the validity of specific products (Perry and Dawson 1985).

In the United States, initial contemplation of such regulation began in the 1880s when the first true food and drug legislation was introduced to Congress. The Pure Food and Drug Act came into effect in 1906, supposedly to protect the public from 'evil scoundrels' trying to make a dollar (Mintz 1985, 113). It was not until 1938 that the FDA had the power to regulate devices for the first time. The definition of a 'device,' which included IUDs, also covered various other items such as electric belts, quack diagnostic scales, bathroom weight scales, shoulder braces, air conditioners, and crutches (Mintz 1985). The FDA could regulate these devices only after they had been out in the medical or public market. Only if numerous reports suggested that a drug or device was dangerous to public health could the FDA step in and take it off the market (Perry and Dawson 1985). However, the rules governing non-medicated devices and medicated devices differed.

In the 1970s non-medicated devices were not under such stringent rules as medicated devices. Because of the construction of the Dalkon Shield, it initially was labelled a non-medicated device. At this time, non-medicated devices did not have to be approved in an official capacity. Because of the absence of certain definitions in the regulations, devices such as the Dalkon Shield escaped scrutiny prior to being released to the public in 1970. This is how the Shield crossed geographical borders.

Because of mounting evidence of improprieties, the U.S. government began to move towards tighter regulations. Only after years of debate in Congress and multiple reports of injuries from the use of the Dalkon Shield was a new law established for premarket regulatory standards for devices. The FDA finally created a Medical Devices Bureau to determine the safety and efficacy of these devices. Not until February 1973 did the FDA establish the regulation that 'IUDs with active ingredients were classified as drugs; those without were devices' (Perry and Dawson 1985, 133). Thus, IUDs containing copper or other active ingredients would be categorized as medicated devices or drugs.

In Canada, a Medical Devices Bureau would not be established until 1978. This bureau is now part of the Health Protection Branch of Health Canada (HPB). However, premarket evaluation within the HPB became established only in 1982. As a result, all IUDs in Canada and the United States now have to pass premarket evaluation.

It is unfortunate that such regulations were not in place when Dr Hugh Davis became interested in developing IUDs. A Johns Hopkins gynecologist, Davis was revered as a physician with an impeccable reputation. His association with the distinguished university placed him in the forefront of the medical field. He was also a man of many ideas, and it seems that one of his aims was to achieve notoriety for the invention of an IUD contraceptive. The Dalkon Shield was not the only device that he would invent. In 1964, Davis and Dr Edmond Jones developed an IUD called the Incon Ring. By 1966 approximately 3,000 Baltimore women were fitted with the Incon. Once again problems developed: the Incon caused uterine perforation (Mintz 1985), and had a high rate of expulsion and failure as a contraceptive. Naturally, these results decreased its marketability. As a result, Ortho Pharmaceutical Company, the product manufacturer, chose not to continue marketing it. This IUD never made it to the open market (Perry and Dawson 1985).

In 1966 a flurry of interest developed over two new patented IUDs: the Lippes Loop and the Saf-T-Coil. Reports on these IUDs first surfaced at a Population Council conference in 1962 (Perry and Dawson 1985; Mintz 1985). These two devices seemed to encourage a positive view of IUDs among the medical and scientific communities. Around the same time that the Lippes Loop and the Saf-T-Coil emerged as viable new contraceptives, the birth control pill also was popular, although as early as the late 1960s the pill's reputation began to decline (Seaman 1969).

This was a period of social and economic change, and the use of safe contraceptives became paramount to many women and couples. Couples wanted to delay starting a family until they had a secure financial footing. Many physicians went along with providing what they believed to be safe contraception to their patients.

Dr Hugh Davis took advantage of these developments in his newfound relationship with Irwin 'Win' Lerner, an electrical engineer. Lerner had a history of working in medical laboratories. Davis and Lerner, along with Robert E. Cohn, Lerner's attorney, formed Lerner Laboratories. In 1967, Davis patented his new IUD. 'In shape it resembled a policeman's badge, which is why it came to be called a Shield' (Mintz 1985). After it was patented, Davis asked Lerner if he could add something to the structure of the device to help secure it in the uterus. Lerner then introduced the ten blunt lateral fins that ran along the sides of the dime-shaped structure. Its shape then resembled a crab-like creature with claws.

Interestingly, when Lerner added the fins to the design of the Shield he then had it patented under his name in 1968, with Davis's full agreement (Mintz 1985). Davis accepted a 5 per cent share of net sales. Provision of clinical testing facilities at Johns Hopkins University were also included in the deal for Lerner. Once sales increased and the three formed a partnership, Davis negotiated a 35 per cent share of the profits. In 1969 the threesome renamed the company Dalkon Corporation. It was at this point that Davis began to promote the Shield as being 99.5 per cent safe, making it a dream contraceptive for many. This promise seemed to have a strong impact on buyers: how could the medical and consumer communities resist a contraceptive that purported to have an almost 100 per cent safety factor?

Davis's promotional rhetoric was initially aimed at physicians. Prestigious American academic journals accepted his reports as valid. They

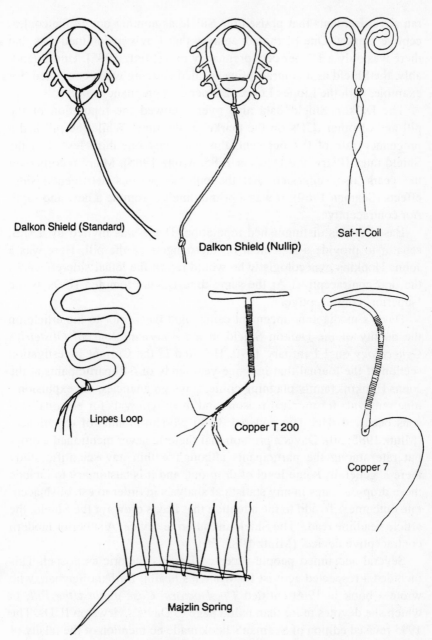

Figure 1. Examples of typical intrauterine devices

ran advertisements that praised the Shield as number one in the contraceptive market. One of the advantages that Davis maintained was that there was only a 1.1 per cent pregnancy rate (Mintz 1985). Understandably, the Shield as a contraceptive seemed enticing when compared, for example, with the Lippes Loop's 2.7 per cent pregnancy rate.

The Dalkon Shield data also overshadowed the reputation of the pill and of other IUDs on the market at the time. While the pill had a pregnancy rate of 0.7 per cent, this was only one-third less than the Shield rates (Perry and Dawson 1985; Mintz 1985). Many reports over the years also suggested that the pill had serious detrimental side-effects (Seaman 1969). It was a prime time to promote a new and superior contraceptive.

Based on his distinguished reputation, Davis was invited by a U.S. senator to provide a statement on the dangers of the pill. Here was a Johns Hopkins gynecologist who would report the lethal side-effects of the oral contraceptive. At the same time Davis promoted IUDs as the 'superior' contraceptive.

Davis's media announcement came eight days prior to his article on the quality of the Dalkon Shield in the *American Journal Obstetrics Gynecology* on 1 February 1970. He cited in the Current Investigation section of the journal that in a one-year study of 640 participants at the Johns Hopkins family planning clinic, 'Five pregnancies, ten expulsions, nine removals for medical reasons and three removals for personal reasons occurred. His data covered 3,549 woman-months of experience' (Mintz 1985, 30). Davis's promotional rhetoric never mentioned a drop-out rate among the participants although within any scientific study there is generally some level of drop-out, and it is customary to include these drop-out rates in any statistical analysis in order to establish accurate outcomes. To add to the attention that Davis drew for the Shield, the article headline read, 'The Shield intrauterine device: A superior modern contraceptive device' (Mintz 1985, 30).

Several acclaimed people accepted Davis's rhetoric as gospel. This included a respected activist for women's health, Barbara Seaman, who wrote a book in 1969 entitled *The Doctors' Case against the Pill*, in which she devotes more than half a page to Davis's views on IUDs. The 1995 revised edition of Seaman's book made no mention of the falsity of Davis's figures. In both editions, Davis is quoted as saying 'the Dalkon

Shield has made many a new bride happy' (169). Davis also promoted his IUD as suitable for all women. In fact, it was not suitable for women who had never been pregnant because of the high risk of PID (Tatum 1975a, 1976, 1977).

Not everyone was seduced by Davis's reports, though. James P. Duffy III, then a minority (Republican) staff counsel, questioned Davis about a patented device that he had registered in his name (Mintz 1985). Davis sidestepped the issue by stating that he did not hold a recent patent on an IUD. He further explained that he had given up ownership of a former patent on the Incon IUD device to Johns Hopkins. 'For a fleeting moment the searchlight beam of publicity had shone on the dark secret of his financial stake in the Dalkon Shield – a secret on which much depended' (Mintz 1985, 37). Davis's statement was accurate, but misleading. His co-ownership of the Dalkon Corporation was a well-hidden fact because he was, in some respects, a silent partner. It was Irwin Lerner who was actually registered as the owner of the Dalkon Shield patent (Mintz 1985). This was typical of Davis and only one of the many clever responses that he provided when questioned about his association with the Dalkon Shield.

By now four partners comprised the Dalkon Corporation: Irwin Lerner, electrical engineer; Dr Hugh Davis; Robert Cohn, lawyer; and Dr Thad Earl. Earl was a medical director of a family planning agency in Defiance, Ohio. He would play an integral role in the ultimate sale of the Shield to A.H. Robins.

When Earl first heard about the Shield he was impressed primarily by the reports of its low pregnancy rate. In addition, he favoured the idea that it was considered a safe contraceptive for women who had never been pregnant. He was also impressed with the ease with which the Shield was inserted into the uterus, as demonstrated by Hugh Davis. As a measure of goodwill, Davis provided Earl with forty-eight samples to take back to his family planning agency. On 8 or 9 December 1969, Earl was the first physician outside of Maryland to implant the Shield in his patients. He would also be the first to encounter problems with it (Mintz 1985). In the beginning, however, he was convinced that the device had a 'great future' (Mintz 1985, 39). Earl further explored the idea of the device with the partners of Dalkon Corporation. In April, he invested $50,000 in the company and thus became its fourth partner (Mintz

1985). Earl would prove to be an exemplary salesperson. Davis, however, seemed to feel that Earl's salesmanship resembled a 'snake oil approach' and 'would turn many people off' (Mintz, 1985, p. 40).

When the Robins company came onto the scene, the Shield's reputation was well above that of all other IUDs. A.H. Robins bought the Dalkon Shield from Dalkon Corporation in approximately 1970 (Mintz 1985). This purchase was based on several factors.

John McClure, an A.H. Robins sales representative, met Thad Earl at a convention in Bedford, Pennsylvania, in May 1970. After McClure talked with Earl and read material on the Shield, he was sufficiently impressed to ask whether the device was for sale. Earl responded positively to the inquiry, but at the same time told McClure that there was another offer in negotiation. Upjohn Corporation had offered the Dalkon Corporation $500,000, plus 6 per cent in royalty interest on future sales of the Shield (Perry and Dawson 1985). Earl told McClure, however, that if he could convince the Robins people to make a better offer, it would be taken into consideration.

A week later, Roy Smith, Director of Product Planning for A.H. Robins, called Thad Earl and arranged a meeting. At the same time, Earl suggested that Smith bring a physician with him, presumably as an expert on IUDs.

Earl and Lerner provided various demonstrations for Roy Smith, Dr Ed Davis (no relation to Hugh Davis), and Dr Frederick Clark as part of the promotional package. As a further means of promoting the Shield, Earl demonstrated its insertion on volunteer patients. He also proudly used his own voice-over to describe the insertion procedures shown in a film. The film had no sound track, and any pain experienced by the patient was not evident to the viewers.

Ed Davis took an immediate dislike to Thad Earl. He felt that Earl was arrogant and self-serving (Perry and Dawson 1985). However, in the final analysis, Ed Davis made his decision about the Shield based on Hugh Davis's original twelve-month study. Weeks later, A.H. Robins made an offer of $750,000 cash and 10 per cent of sales to Dalkon Corporation for the device. As part of the package, Robins also invited Davis, Lerner, and Earl to join the company as consultants (Perry and Dawson 1985).

Several top executives within Robins were confident that the

Shield held promise for increasing Robins's profits. Indeed they were right. During the national marketing campaign, Lerner supervised the assembling, packaging, and shipping of the Shield to Robins. With this arrangement, Lerner sold each device to Robins for 35 cents. Robins then sold each device to physicians for $4. In turn, the physicians sold it to North American patients for approximately $12. At least four million of these devices were sold worldwide (Perry and Dawson 1985).

Still, some members of Robins expressed scepticism about the device. George Thomas, vice-president of Robin's international division, wrote a memo about his concerns to William Zimmer, executive vice-president and chief operating officer, 'I worry that we seem to have no present or past R&D [research and development] effort on contraception and contraceptive methods ... I worry about the fact that we have no market knowledge or experience in our company' (Perry and Dawson 1985, 62–63). His concerns were ultimately ignored.

Knowledge of potential problems with the Dalkon Shield spread throughout the corporation. Robins's management knew the Shield had a higher pregnancy rate than originally projected by Davis. At this point, it was projected more in the range of 3.1 per cent, not the earlier 1.1 per cent. Later this estimate would grow to 5–6 per cent. Further warnings came from Lerner, of all people (Mintz 1985).

Most IUDs have a monofilament string (a single thread). Unfortunately, when tested, the monofilament string of the Dalkon Shield had a tendency to break. Thus, A.H. Robins's executives decided that a multi-filament string covered with an open-ended sheath would provide the best security against both breakage and infection. However, an executive of Chapstick, a Robins subsidiary, 'left a coated tail in a beaker of water one day, and watched with fascination as droplets gradually travelled from the tip to the top' (Fido and Fido 1996, 124). Dr Howard Tatum had observed a similar phenomenon.

Lerner urged that the multifilament string be tested for a possible wicking effect (Perry and Dawson 1985). As a result, Dr Fletcher Owen, a Robins employee, was designated to examine possible defects of the tail string. The extent of his examination was a review of literature on IUD strings. Owen then reported that there was no literature on multifilament strings. The result of Owen's review was that Robins failed to do any official wicking or safety tests on the string in the four years they had the Shield on the market. The construction of the string became one of the main issues of contention associated with the problems of the Dalkon Shield.

Around the same time, Hugh Davis also pressured the company to make changes to the Shield. Davis foresaw trouble from the FDA if copper was not added to the Shield. 'Copper is thought to inhibit bacterial growth and decrease chances of pregnancy' (Tatum 1977, 8). The addition of copper would place the Shield in a drug category with the FDA. It would also help to decrease the reported pregnancy rate among users of the Shield. The suggested changes worried the Robins group at the time, but apparently not enough. In a further effort to avoid problems, Davis also wanted the width of the Shield to be reduced from 27 to 24 mm (Perry and Dawson 1985); he felt that this would help reduce cramping and bleeding. Davis then suggested that the fins be made more 'bat-like'; this, he said, would reduce the expulsion rate. It is interesting to note that Davis and Lerner would choose this time to suggest these changes to Robins; it was possible that they feared the new FDA regulations.

Robins was reluctant to make the changes because it meant the new dimensions would not conform to Davis's original study. This naturally meant that additional testing should be conducted. It also meant time and money. Robins went ahead with the changes anyway, but continued promoting the Dalkon Shield based on Davis's original data (Perry and Dawson 1985). As time went on, several company executives expressed concern about this: Wayne Crowder, C.E. Moreton, Roy Smith, Bob Nickless, Ernest Bender, and others. At this point, all of these men knew of the potential problems with the device. Again, concerns extended from the validity of Davis's original study to the composition of the Shield itself and its multifilament string.

Questions that arose about various aspects of the Shield from internal staff, along with proposed changes in FDA regulations, increased the push for publicity for the Shield in the medical and public domains.

The widespread destructiveness of the Dalkon Shield began when advertisements carried the same inaccurate data that Davis and others had previously used to seduce consumers, who included physicians and patients. Information disseminated by A.H. Robins about the supposed 'superiority' of the Shield aimed to attract as many buyers as possible.

In fact, the publicity campaign created through Wilcox and Williams Public Relations Agency succeeded in selling great numbers of the device. 'In January 1971, 29,000 Shields had been inserted. In June, the monthly insertion rate had more than doubled to 66,000' (Perry and Dawson 1985, 72). Sales of all IUDs within the United States in 1971 reached an all-time high of 1,670,000. Approximately two million American women and 123,000 Canadian women ultimately were persuaded to buy the Shield through their physician or from family planning clinics. The remaining Shields were sold to women in developing countries.

Advertisements and articles in women's magazines encouraged women to 'protect' themselves with the Shield. The remaining female world population heard of the Shield through their physicians or from family planning clinics and the U.S. Agency for International Development (AID).

Advertisements placed in several medical journals such as the *American Journal Obstetrics Gynecology* (1971–72) and the *Journal of Reproductive Medicine* (1972–73) aimed to sell the device to physicians. The 'lay ads,' or public ads that targeted women, and in some respects their spouses, broke specific pharmaceutical ethical codes. At the time, such advertising tactics were prohibited in public magazines. (This same strategy was later used by some lawyers to recruit clients who had used the device.) According to Baltimore lawyer Mike Pretl, 'There was an issue of a mini-scandal, if I can call it that, of 'lay' advertising because it was ... and to a lesser extent still is considered unethical under the pharmaceutical manufacturers code of good practices to run promotional materials in 'lay' magazines. But we were able to establish that Robins had paid some PR people to write articles which they then planted in *Redbook* and *Family Circle* and *Woman's Day* and magazines like that, talking about this 'great' new IUD. That is considered borderline unethical under the code ... I suspect a lot of companies were doing that' (M. Pretl, interview, 18 December 1995).

Pretl later went on to explain that Robins spent millions on promoting the device through Wilcox and Williams. In the fall of 1971, Robins hired the Manhattan PR firm to create an aggressive publicity campaign to sell the Dalkon Shield. The firm's president, Richard Wilcox, proposed a campaign based on information sent to him by Richard Velz of Robins's public relations division. Wilcox suggested that they stimulate the interest of editors of major women's magazines. The campaign would target women through such magazines as *Ladies' Home Journal*, *Mademoiselle,* and *Family Circle.*

Velz wrote a memo to then vice-president of Robins, Dr Jack Freund: 'As you know, Mr Robins has assigned top priority to special promotion of the Dalkon Shield in other than medical and trade magazines' (Mintz 1985, 90–91). At the time, some articles written for magazines had to be monitored to avoid similar content in more than one magazine. In fact, an article prepared by Davis that had been previously shelved by one of the popular magazines years earlier was pulled and revamped for a possible run in the spring of 1972. Earl also submitted a story to a magazine. Subsequently, Velz expressed his concern that the whole program could be put in jeopardy if 'order' was not applied to the submission of information to magazines. Soon after, arrangements for any publicity had to be run through Wilcox and Williams; they would oversee the overall campaign (Mintz 1985). This establishment of order launched the initial steps of what would become a windfall for A.H. Robins.

It seems that Wilcox and Williams Agency may have been another victim of the lies and deceit of Davis and Robins. The data sent to the PR firm reproduced the figures and percentages of Davis's original study. Two months prior to the launch of the publicity campaign, Frederick Clark, a Robins official, expressed concern over the lack of testing of the new Dalkon Shield. He suggested that some sort of information be on file to respond to questions from physicians, and he urged testing for this purpose. However, 'observations' by one or two investigators were all that apparently constituted the premarket testing (Perry and Dawson 1985).

Likewise, a warning of misrepresentation of the Shield in advertisements was sent to various staff at A.H. Robins via an internal memo. Allen Polon, Project Coordinator, sent it to Bob Hogsett, Manager of Promotional Services, with copies to John Burke, Kitty Preston, Dale Taylor, Roger Tuttle, Alan Young, Frank Mann, George Thomas, and Arthur Cummings, all top managers in the company. The memo stated, in part,

This memo is referencing two pieces of Dalkon Shield advertising literature which you questioned me about. The first is the 8 page advertisement titled 'A.H. Robins – A Progress Report – The IUD that's changing current thinking about contraceptives ...' In this advertisement a table is entitled, 'Clinical Results to Date' which is outdated and parts of which are no longer valid ... The other advertisement in question is the earlier 2 page ad with a large picture in the foreground of a uterus with the Dalkon Shield inserted. This, too, is out of date for two reasons. A pregnancy rate of 1.1% is stated which is not valid and the labeling at the bottom of the second page is incomplete and no longer used. Therefore, please do not continue to use the two advertisements ... (Polon 1973)

In response, the A.H. Robins company never told the medical profession of the FDA and certainly not the Public, that its Dalkon Shield project coordinator had repudiated the claims with which it had induced physicians to implant the devices in millions of women (Mintz 1985, 83). Several advertisements made false claims about the 'superiority' of the Dalkon Shield despite numerous warnings to Robins staff. Despite the memo and these false claims, the company continued to market the Dalkon Shield.

The CEOs and President E. Clairborne Robins, Jr, knew that they had just promoted a bad product to the medical and patient community (Perry and Dawson 1985; Mintz 1985). Plastics toxicologist Dr John Autian suggested to Robins executives that a time period be placed on the use of the Dalkon Shield because it had a 'definite problem with this [nylon string]' (Mintz 1985, 137). Autian maintained that historically it had been shown that nylon deteriorates over a period of time. Despite his recommendations, Robins 'armed its salesmen with a new competitive tool by telling them to note that we no longer recommend replacement of the Dalkon Shield every two years"' (Mintz 1985, 138). In fact, 'For eight years Robins ... persisted in claiming that a nonpregnant woman could continue to use the Shield safely unless symptoms of infection appeared' (Mintz 1985, 137–38). All those who actively participated in providing the information for the advertisements had apparently colluded to deceive the medical community and the patient population.

Others who knew felt paralysed, and were divided about whether to challenge the hierarchy and risk losing their jobs. Wayne Crowder, quality control supervisor for Robins, feared his job was threatened. In fact, he was instructed by another Robins employee to 'leave it alone.' Ultimately, he was fired for speaking out (Mintz 1985). Crowder, like some others, felt confused and betrayed by the company when it did not heed his warnings early in the process that the tail string of the device had wicking problems (Mintz 1985). Dr Howard Tatum, formerly with the Population Council, was concerned about reports of problems with the Dalkon Shield. He decided to test it himself. He suspended the tail string of the Dalkon Shield along with other IUD strings in a dye. With the Dalkon Shield string, the dye climbed the length of the string and through the two knots. Tatum revealed that the multifilament string of the IUD contained viable-appearing bacteria within the sheath between the fibres (Tatum 1977). The others had a monofilament string and did not respond in the same way. Tatum's suspicions, along with Crowder's, were confirmed: the string wicked. Again, their advice was not heeded. Unfortunately, many such warnings passed over the heads of others at A.H. Robins. Tatum went to the FDA with his findings.

A worst-case scenario is depicted in Karen Hicks's 1994 book *Surviving the Dalkon Shield*, in which she describes how Frances Cleary's father-in-law, Robert Nickless, then Robins's vice-president of international marketing, knowingly advocated the Shield to his daughter-in-law. Frances Cleary later incurred severe pain from pelvic inflammatory disease and underwent surgery. She did not realize her father-in-law's betrayal until the publicity surrounding the dangers of the Shield became public around 1985. By this time, her father-in-law had died. Cleary later discovered the extent of his involvement through Morton Mintz's 1985 book *At Any Cost*. This scenario was only one among many acts of betrayal surrounding the Dalkon Shield. Ironically, many people were either convinced of the Shield's excellence or of its dangers through similar media: journal articles, magazine advertisements, or television news.

Target audiences were betrayed by equally persuasive messages through some of the imagery used in the advertisements. Messages conveying the dehumanization of women through fragmentation of their internal bodies were sometimes blatant, sometimes more subtle. One of the most degrading advertisements placed in medical journals during 1970–71 came to be known as the Flying Uterus to plaintiff lawyers. It showed what looked to be a rubber uterus with a Dalkon Shield inserted in it, along with various oddly shaped smaller uteri floating in the background in a cloudy sky. Tiny pollywog faces or distorted images of ovaries also seemed to emerge on either side of the artificial uterus. Author and activist Karen Hicks describes the imagery as follows: 'Other symbols in the background of the advertisement include what appears to be an engineering calibration tool, as well as other floating uteri, impaled on a backdrop of scientific chart grids' (Hicks 1994, 31).

Other such advertisements projected tamer images; however, the degrading rhetoric in the text conveyed an image of women as either disorganized, depressed, or reactionary. One headline described 'The Nullip,' 'The Pill Reactor,' 'The Clinic Patient,' and 'The Disorganized Woman.' The last paragraph in this advertisement promised the physician that he or she was presenting an offering to the patient. Women were promised protection even from themselves: 'With the Dalkon Shield the patient can throw away her calendars, charts, and dispensers ... She makes just one decision – to have the Dalkon Shield inserted. From this moment on, she is protected 24 hours a day' (1971).

Another advertisement headline read, 'Before 1970, IUDs were seldom considered as a contraceptive method of first choice. The Dalkon Shield is changing that.' Ironically, the events surrounding the failures of the Shield have in fact contributed to the decreased use of IUDs in the 1990s.

Further advertisements used manipulative rhetoric to gain the confidence of their audience. Words such as 'secret' and 'high degree of ... effectiveness' may have appealed to the observers' thinking in that they felt they were getting something special. Terms such as 'ingenious' again suggested something unique; for example, 'What is the secret of the Dalkon Shield's high degree of contraceptive effectiveness? The answer lies in its ingenious design.' This ad displayed a silicone mould of a uterine cavity created by Hugh Davis and Robert Israel as a prototype for devising measurements for the Dalkon Shield design. To the right of this lay an image of a real uterine cavity; the text alongside it stated: Note optimum fit of Dalkon Shield to configuration of the uterine cavity. Unique fin design provides "fundus-seeking" effect when uterus contracts, one of the factors which contributes to the Shield's extremely low expulsion rate.' It would not be surprising if the expulsion rate was low, since the 'unique fins' gripped the uterus. Moreover, physicians often expressed concern about the 'unique fins' because of their propensity to tear the uterus and cervix upon withdrawal of the Shield.

The Shield was first promoted primarily to general practitioners, osteopaths, and obstetricians-gynecologists. Its simplicity, flexibility, and convenience initially impressed most physicians. Nevertheless, many expressed scepticism upon first sight of the Dalkon Shield. The crochet needle–like inserter concerned them because of the high risk of perforation to the uterus; the fins looked like sharp teeth that could tear the uterus and cervix if manoeuvred inaccurately. They also knew that the Shield caused a great deal of pain for the patient upon insertion.

Ultimately, negative reports about frequent infection for women using the Dalkon Shield started to flood the Robins offices. Despite meetings with upper management, the problem was not monumental enough to them to worry about (Perry and Dawson 1985). These factors, along with lack of instruction or practice in inserting the device, made physicians uneasy. As a result, some completely rejected the device; others, despite their reservations, went on to implant thousands of Dalkon Shields into unsuspecting patients.

Much of the physicians' training had been derived from viewing films about the insertion process, clinical demonstrations, brochures, or through detail representatives (sales representatives). The job of these representatives was to provide 'detailed' information to the physician about a particular product. During the 1970s, these young men and women, who often were not medically trained, were hired to promote the Shield. Usually, warnings of any high risk of potential damage were written in small print on the Dalkon Shield package. More often than not, these packages were not read before being tossed into the garbage.

Finally, a common outcome of the use of IUDs is an increased risk of pelvic inflammatory disease (PID), which may be followed by infertility (Vessey, et al. 1983). For those who became pregnant, many did not go to full term.

One might ask why, if there were similar problems with IUDs in general, was there such extensive litigation around the Dalkon Shield? According to Baltimore lawyer Mike Pretl, 'The numbers of women injured and the lies and deceit that arose from the events surrounding the Dalkon Shield brought it into the public realm!' (M. Pretl, interview, 18 December 1995).

When Pretl was asked if Hugh Davis had any conscience about his part in the Dalkon Shield saga, Pretl said, 'I've taken several depositions from Davis and he maintained that it's never been proven that his Shield caused all these problems ... I think he believed that ... but one of the things you learn in litigation is that everybody has a personal defense mechanism that lets them justify themselves and you marshal the facts that support you [such as] "God Damn it's just these lawyers that are try-ing to make money" ... but, a lot of good physicians feel that way, too, ... that most malpractice is trumped up litigation' (M. Pretl, interview, 18 December 1995).

Without a doubt, the human costs incurred from the imperfections of the Shield are great. Nevertheless, there still remains uncertainty among the medical community about the problems caused by the use of IUDs, specifically the Dalkon Shield. Because of this uncertainty, there has been a marked decrease in the sale of IUDs in North America in the 1990s compared with other contraceptive methods.

Physicians such as Dr Norman Barwin, Dr Dorothy Shaw, and Dr Brian Ivey, among other physicians interviewed for this book, reiterate that the litigation surrounding the Dalkon Shield has downgraded the image of all IUDs, perhaps unfairly. In fact, they still maintain that some IUDs provide a viable contraceptive means. Today, many physicians concede that women must research the side-effects of IUDs and consult two or three doctors to determine whether this form of contraceptive is for them.

There are countless details related to the events just described; how-ever, the first two chapters of this book are intended to provide only a brief overview of the background issues of the Dalkon Shield saga. Further details can be found in Morton Mintz's book *At Any Cost: Cor-porate Greed, Women, and the Dalkon Shield* (1985); Susan Perry and Jim Dawson's *Nightmare: Women and the Dalkon Shield* (1985); Nicole Grant's *Selling of Contraception* (1992); Richard Sobol's *Bend-ing the Law: The Story of the Dalkon Shield Bankruptcy* (1991); and Dr Karen Hicks's *Surviving the Dalkon Shield IUD: Women v. the Pharmaceutical Industry* (1994). These books provide detailed perspectives of the legal, political, and sociological aspects of the Dalkon Shield story.

The remaining chapters of this book will provide a comprehensive and in-depth examination of the human cost for the diverse players in this story. Much of the information to follow is gathered from those who had firsthand experience with the Shield in some way.

2

Greed, Deceit, and Non-accountability

It is more than twenty years (1971–74) since four million women world-wide used the Dalkon Shield. Many of these women incurred irreversible damage to their reproductive organs, losing their natural right to motherhood as a consequence. Their spouses also lost their right to share in the creation of a new life. Single women's prospects for marriage became limited owing to their inability to conceive or to carry a child to full term. Thus, all the players linked with the Dalkon Shield incurred grave human costs.

Ivy Tremaine of Quebec gave birth to a child who had the imprint of the Shield on the side of its skull. Nancy Campbell of British Columbia underwent numerous operations due to pelvic inflammatory disease; ultimately she had no choice but to have an unwanted hysterectomy. Karen Hicks of Pennsylvania experienced seven years of excruciating pain. A series of doctors told her she was neurotic and unbalanced. 'Finally, in 1978, a new gynecologist removed the device, but [Hicks] continued to be ill, she had no energy, her marriage broke up' (Stewart 1995, 173–74). She married again in 1984, but 'infection persisted; she then reluctantly agreed to have a complete hysterectomy ... it was at this time that her doctor told her that her problems may be incurred from the Dalkon Shield' (Stewart 1995, 173–74). Pauline Belanger of Alberta experienced a premature birth due to the rampant infection throughout her body. The Dalkon Shield remained in place during her pregnancy. Pauline and the baby girl both suffered severe infection. The child, named Solange, died in an incubator after five days of fighting for her life. Pauline said she saw Solange for the last time about half an hour before she died: 'I knew that she was crossing over. She opened her eyes, and looked at me. This is the only time that she opened her eyes ... sometimes when I think of her looking at me, I find the pain unbearable. I want to scream and rage, and curse this world in which babies die' (P. Belanger, correspondence, 1995). Gerry wept as he related the story of the loss of his son. His wife had miscarried at five months because of problems that developed from an embedded Shield (see Appendix B). Many such examples led women and some of their spouses worldwide to take a public stand against A.H. Robins Company and its insurers.

Between 1978 and 1995, numerous individuals and groups filed class action and individual lawsuits against Robins. Many lawyers and judges became involved in the hundreds of thousands of lawsuit proceedings. Years of controversy have surrounded the use of the Dalkon Shield, effectively dividing medical, legal, family, family planning groups, and consumer activist groups. Such divisions extend to the present day and have produced unsettling consequences for the players linked one way or another to the making, marketing, and removal of the Dalkon Shield.

One of the many consequences of the Dalkon Shield saga, apart from injury to women, includes a citizens' class action lawsuit by the U.S. National Women's Health Network, which filed a court action against Robins in 1981 and petitioned the U.S. Food and Drug Administration in 1983, seeking a worldwide recall of the Dalkon Shield. 'Although unsuccessful, the lawsuit provided an important means of educating the public' (Boston Women's Health Book Collective 1994, p. 294). The lawsuit also encouraged others to take a stand against Robins. For some, the success of further lawsuits held out at least some hope of recognition for a wrong committed against unknowing victims.

In a separate case in 1986 Glenda Breland and many other claimants filed suit against Aetna Casualty and Surety Company, Robins's product liability insurer. Preceding Robins's reorganization of its assets, this was a class action on behalf of all persons injured by the Dalkon Shield (Mintz 1985; Sobol 1991; Hicks 1994; U.S. Bankruptcy Court 1988). Under the settlement, Aetna would provide additional insurance coverage for Dalkon Shield claims. This insurance would be distributed to the claimants under what would become the Robins bankruptcy plan (U.S. Bankruptcy Court 1988).

In 1978 Aetna moved to release itself from having to renew liability insurance for Robins. This, in turn, created a dispute between Aetna and Robins. The dispute focused on how much the insurance company should be required to pay in Dalkon Shield cases. Would settlements be calculated from the time a woman had the Shield inserted or from the time she incurred injury? This was a key point of contention, since it alluded to a time at which Aetna undoubtedly knew of the alleged problems with the Shield. If the company's role as insurer stemmed from the time women had the IUD inserted, then they would have to pay a much higher monetary contribution for claimants' awards. Robins argued that Aetna's involvement stemmed from the time women had the Shield inserted.

Robins and Aetna fought it out in the courts for approximately four years. In 1984, Aetna agreed to provide '$70 million to its coverage of the Shield, bringing the total amount of insurance money available from Aetna for Shield litigation to 369 million' (Perry and Dawson 1985, 238). The agreement to pay proved interesting in that it implied collusion between Aetna and Robins, suggesting that Aetna was aware of the alleged problems with the Shield from the time when Robins initially purchased the Shield in 1970 (Mintz 1985).

Before an agreement between Aetna and Robins could be consummated, the well-publicized civil action suits against Aetna involving Glenda Breland, et al. (November 1986) needed final closure. 'In order for the settlement between Robins and Aetna to be binding, it [was] necessary that the Court approve the settlement and dismissal of the Breland case' (U.S. Bankruptcy Court 1988). The remaining Breland claims under the new agreement meant the said claimants would receive similar options to those under the Claimants Trust Fund. Prior to this settlement agreement, 'In 1983 Laureen Ford won a 4.9 million dollar award in Dade Circuit Court against Robins. Ford's award was the second largest monetary settlement awarded' (Arocha 1983, front page). 'The highest amount went to a Colorado woman who claimed she became sterile because of the Dalkon Shield. She was awarded 6.8 million dollars' (Mintz 1985, 149–50). Carie Palmer of Kansas received $600,000 in compensatory damages and $6.2 million in punitive damages. These

awards represented monetary compensation for the physical and emotional damage she incurred from the Shield. At this point in the litigation
history, A.H. Robins had already lost several cases involving the IUD,
according to company officials (Arocha 1983; Mintz 1985). At that
time, Robins appealed some of the awards.

Aetna routinely resorted to questionable tactics to defend its position.
Depositions taken from women suing Aetna and Robins included insen-
sitive and degrading questions about their personal hygiene and sex
lives. 'The record shows that Robins' attorneys took depositions from
Shield victims in which they asked not only intimate, but also demean-
ing and even intimidating questions' (Mintz 1985, 194). The implications were that these women had not contracted pelvic inflammatory
disease from the Dalkon Shield, but rather as a result of promiscuous
behaviour and unhygienic habits (Mintz 1985). The same attitude was
reflected in claim forms that asked women to account for their sexual
history.

The fact that these tactics were being used incensed those who knew
that they reflected how far the companies were willing to go to avoid
accountability. What A.H. Robins failed to see, according to Laura
Jones, then a Vancouver consumer activist, is that 'This is not just about
women, but their spouses, boyfriends, children and grandparents'
('Dalkon: A contraceptive ...' 1988, B5). Some women's sense of well-
being was also challenged by their physicians: 'Instead of identifying
the women's problem, doctors treated them like hypochondriacs or,
worse, implied they were promiscuous for contracting pelvic inflammatory disease' ('Dalkon: A contraceptive ...' 1988, B5).

A.H. Robins filed a petition with the U.S. Bankruptcy Court in
August 1985 for protection under Chapter 11 of the U.S. Bankruptcy
Code (Hicks 1994, 6). Judge Robert Merhige Jr agreed. A reorganization plan was submitted to the Court in February 1988, which was confirmed by Judge Merhige at a hearing on 19 July 1988. Under Chapter
11, a company is allowed to reoganize its assets and come up with a plan
to pay its debt, in this case, to the Dalkon Shield claimants. Even though
Merhige appeared anxious to resolve the case by helping all involved,
200,000 claimants and ten lawyers representing them moved to have
him disqualified from the case in March 1986. Primarily, the lawyers
felt that Merhige's alleged personal friendship with E. Clairborne Rob-

ins, Sr (retired, but still a major shareholder in the company) and his financial and legal relationships with Richmond, Virginia, lawyers representing parties in the case was not appropriate (Courie 1986). Further, according to various sources Merhige lived down the street from E. Clairborne Robins, Jr (Stewart 1995). Despite this fact, Merhige denied that Robins was a friend, but described him as a 'fine man' (Stewart 1995, 197).

Not surprisingly, negative publicity surrounding Robins's difficulties 'caused the price of a share of Robins' stock to fall to $8 from a 1985 high of over $24, and one that made most every front page in the country' (Mintz 1985, 245). This did not discourage many offers from other corporations to buy Robins, but American Home Products (AHP), a Delaware company, provided the best terms of agreement.

Robins's reorganization plan proposed that it would establish a safe and fair means for claimants to receive monetary compensation. The plan was also proposed as a means to an end for the company. In total, approximately $3 billion was paid to Robins through its merger with AHP. Some of this merger money was split among various sources. For example, Robins and its stockholders walked away with approximately $750 million of American Home Products shares (Canadian Press 1988). This left the rest of the revenue to be placed in a trust fund for the claimants. A feature of the plan is that it made approximately $2.35 billion plus its interest available for Dalkon Shield claims and trust expenses. Robins added another $10 million to the fund to escape further liability related to the Shield, bringing the total amount of the fund to $2.45 billion. Another $50 million went into a second fund to reimburse parties such as doctors and hospitals. These people and organizations would be paid only if they had claims brought directly against them by Dalkon Shield claimants. None of the money in either of the funds could be returned to Robins. In fact, funds left over from the second fund would then be available as direct payment to the claimants. This would later be called the pro rata distribution, by which most claimants would receive, at the end of 1995, another 60 per cent of their original monetary compensation. At the end of 1996, the Dalkon Shield Claimants Trust issued claimants another 25 per cent of their original monetary settlement. At the end of

1999, claimants would receive another 15 per cent pro rata distribution. The Claimants Trust Fund had full responsibility for disseminating awards to claimants, releasing Robins from any further liability.

As a result of the reorganization of Robins's assets, Dalkon Shield claimants became creditors. They had to file claim forms and stand in line to get paid with the trade creditors of the corporation. These women did not receive nearly the amount of monetary compensation as the earlier mentioned cases. Awards ranged from $100 to close to $250,000 for a similar scale of injury.

As New York lawyer Sybil Shainwald explained, 'Corporate America can hide behind Chapter 11 proceedings ... and I am very much opposed to that ... I would rather see them file for Chapter 7 bankruptcy proceedings [see Appendix C] which is "real" bankruptcy ... they [Robins], as you know, were bought out by American Home Products (AHP) ... you know they had to be a profitable company for AHP to buy them' (S. Shainwald, interview, 4 December 1995). However, according to some lawyers representing these cases, the bankruptcy under Chapter 11 allowed foreign claimants to receive similar awards to those of American claimants. In fact, many lawyers encouraged foreign claimants to settle under Robins's reorganization plan because they would ultimately get a better deal. Shainwald continued, 'I agree with this idea [of claimants being discouraged from fighting in the courts for punitive damages] because foreign claimants (this includes Canadians) do not do well in American courts when they sue because the U.S. courts have a doctrine called non-convenience. In a case like this, the courts will say, "This isn't a convenience form, and send the foreigner back home"' (S. Shainwald, interview, 4 December 1995).

Constance Miller, a former Dalkon Shield activist from Seattle, Washington, stated that often the courts would discount foreign claims: 'The sole reason for denying their claims was procedural, according to Miller: the misspelled names delayed the timely receipt of the official questionnaire' (Hicks 1994; 45). Therefore, some foreign claimants missed the deadline through no fault of their own. This appears to be another way in which the administration sidestepped additional claims.

By 1 July 1991, 179,000 American women and 4,000 Canadian women had filed claims. A late claim deadline allowed women who missed the initial deadline of 30 April 1986 to file claims on 30 June

1994. Those who had not yet submitted their complete packet of information were able to gather and submit all of the medical evidence needed to support their claim on 30 June 1995. By 1995, approximately 200,000 Americans and 7,000 Canadians had filed claims. These extended dates allowed additional women an opportunity to receive compensation for their injuries.

Approximately two million American women and 123,000 Canadian women were fitted with the Shield in the 1970s. The remaining women were from all over the world, from places as far flung as Australia, Bangladesh, Thailand, and Brazil (see Appendix E). Although the Dalkon Shield is no longer on the market, Sybil Shainwald notes that she has seen medical evidence of a woman from the United Arab Emirates who had a Shield inserted in 1982. This woman died from infection developed through its use (S. Shainwald, interview, 4 December 1995). Many believe that the Shield continues to be used in developing countries (Boston Women's Health Book Collective 1994). One source indicated that the Shield was promoted to women in developing countries as a viable product simply because it was manufactured in America (Anonymous 1995).

Robins did not appear to be suffering throughout this process. However, the reorganization plan resulted in a legal maze that left claimants feeling isolated from a process that was intended to provide some kind of compensation for their losses. For some, the plan was not acceptable.

Enraged women's outreach groups marched in protest of Robins's attempt to get off the hook. Through the media the women's groups encouraged claimants not to vote for the reorganization plan. For some, the plan would delay the commencement of their payments for two years. Lawyers, for the most part, encouraged women to vote in favour of the plan; others offered to vote on behalf of their clients. Many of the claimants never received the information contained in the report entitled *Sixth Amended and Restated Disclosure Statement* (U.S. Bankruptcy Court 1988), which was a compilation of the details of the final reorganization plan. Thus, often they were not informed well enough to make a decision. As a result, some women went along with their lawyers' 'take charge' action. Other women received only a brief explanation of the plan. With this new development, it seemed the plan would favour only lawyers and Robins's stockholders.

Laura Jones, Elaine Cumley, and four other women continued the activities of Dalkon Shield Action Canada (DSAC), a group that stemmed from the Vancouver Women's Health Collective. Karen Hicks founded the Dalkon Shield Information Network, U.S.A. (DSIN); Belita Cowan founded the National Women's Health Network (NWHN); Rosemary Menard-Sanford and Constance Miller were founding members of the International Dalkon Shield Victims Educational Association (IDEA); and Linda Hightower pioneered the Dalkon Shield Victims (DSV). Some of these outreach or activist groups helped women complete claimant forms and establish connections with lawyers. However, some group leaders advocated filing claims directly with the Claimants Trust Fund instead of with a lawyer to avoid legal contingency fees that claimants would later have deducted from their awards. Some of these legal fees ranged from 25 per cent to 50 per cent of the claimants' awards. In other words, if a claimant received $50,000, she might take home only $25,000. Claimants and some lawyers agree that some of the contingency fees escalated to unreasonable amounts.

Several other health collectives established themselves as information providers for the users of the Dalkon Shield. A few of these groups included the Boston Women's Health Book Collective, Birth Control Victims Canada, and the Mauri Spehar Health Collective. Each of these groups had similar agendas in that they aimed to provide information for the women and put a stop to any further injustices towards any person filing a claim with the Trust.

The Trust was an appointed administrative body that allocated funds as well as set specific guidelines for distributing these funds. Michael Sheppard, a former U.S. Bankruptcy Court clerk, was appointed its executive director.

Linda Thomason was appointed general counsel to the Trust. Thomason had previously worked in a Richmond, Virginia, law firm where she had been part of the Robins defence team during the bankruptcy litigation (Hicks 1994). Laura Jones, executive director of Dalkon Shield Action Canada, while at a conference in Richmond, questioned Thomason's reasons for presenting herself as an advocate for the claimants in her position as general counsel for the Trust. Thomason's response was honest: 'Yes I did work with Robins ... I now work with you and I will try to do my best.' As the discussion between Jones and Thomason continued, Michael Sheppard intervened and inquired what they were talking about. Jones later recounted that there seemed to be an air of 'I don't want you talking about past events' (L. Jones, interview, 14 October 1995). This kind of challenge was not uncommon among those dealing with either the people involved or with other aspects of the litigation process. In some respects, it epitomized the general uneasiness felt among the various groups (Hicks 1994).

Judge Merhige initially approved the appointment of five trustees to the Dalkon Shield Claimants Trust Fund. The trustees' main job was to set up the Trust. Their functions resembled those of a corporate board of directors; they received an annuity plus salary for each formal meeting, as well as expenses. 'They set the Trust's policies, approved all the employment decisions regarding all expenditures and investment strategies ... Nevertheless, Merhige retained the supervisory role over all the budgets' (Hicks 1994, 70).

Despite Merhige's initial approval of the trustees, his perspective later took a turn. Three of the trustees had been elected from nominations by the Dalkon Shield Claimants' Committee. Merhige went along with this temporarily, but subsequently targeted these three people. In a hearing he harshly reprimanded all of them, but particularly Ann Samani, saying that she had a confrontational style. Later, he fired all three of them, expressing his displeasure in their decision-making skills and in the slow process of distributing the funds. Merhige replaced two of the trustees with his own appointees. Earlier, on 4 March 1986, he had fired the original thirty-eight-member Claimants' Committee composed of lawyers, saying they were indecisive about their commitment to cooperating with the bankruptcy (Mintz 1989). At one point, prior to approval of the plan, Merhige was quoted as saying: 'I'm not going to delay this any more ... these women have waited, waited and waited' (Associated Press 1988). It seemed that Merhige operated with an 'iron hand,' yet with an element of compassion for the women.

On 20 March 1986, the United States Trustee appointed a new and smaller Claimants' Committee. Under Chapter 11 procedures committee trustees had to represent people holding Dalkon Shield personal injury claims (Hicks 1994). Representation for the claimants became almost necessary for their sanity because of the perplexing legal intricacies.

The Trust would administer and settle as well as pay claims to separate groups: (1) people who suffered personal injury and eligible members of their families, as well as (2) 'Other' Claimants, including physicians, hospitals, and directors of the company. Those within the 'Other' Claimants group could be compensated if they had been sued themselves in connection with the Dalkon Shield.

Those with personal injury claims could file under one of four options, which were aimed at categorizing the women's claims according to the level of injury they incurred. For example, if a woman's claim rendered her minimally injured, then she would be slotted into Option 1. This option was also for women who could not prove injury because of lost or missing medical records whether they were seriously injured or not. The women in this group were obliged to provide written testimony that they had used the Dalkon Shield, and they could receive only between $100 and $750. In effect, this was a weeding-out process in order that the Trust could concentrate on what were regarded as more 'serious' cases.

Option 2 claimants had to show through medical records that they had used a Dalkon Shield. They did not have to substantiate injury caused by the use of the Shield. Option 3 required affidavits from the claimants stating details of their alleged injuries. The claimants' complete medical records had to be examined in order to show that the injuries were incurred as a result of the Shield and no other IUD. If the settlement offered under this option was not acceptable to a claimant, she could counter the offer. A further stage of in-depth review could also be requested. Option 4 made it possible for women to file claims for injuries that might occur in the future as a result of the Dalkon Shield. Settlements for all four options related to proof of use of the Shield and personal injury. Because monetary compensation was contingent on the alleged extent of injury, it varied substantially. The intricacies of the four options are far more complex than what is described here; however, the complete details are arduous and can be found in other publications that deal with the specifics of this particular process (U.S. Bankruptcy Court 1988; Hicks 1994; Sobol 1991).

The ultimate decision on compensation often depended on the availability of medical records that contained documentation confirming personal injury. Finally, in most cases physicians were asked to retrieve the patients' records from over a ten-year period; a physician then would have to be willing to provide a written confirmation of injury. Physicians often perceived this as risky business, thus 'Women seeking medical records in their fight with Robins have been told they aren't available or had been destroyed ('Dalkon: A contraceptive ...' 1988, B5). In all fairness, though, some of these records may have been missing because in most provinces and states physicians can legally dispose of records after a seven- to ten-year period.

Once the plan was established in 1988, formal notification to potential claimants was disseminated worldwide through various news media. For example, in Canada and the United States a television commercial let claimants know where they could file a claim. It also informed potential claimants that they could deal directly with the Trust instead of going through a lawyer.

In comparison with American claimants, most foreign claimants received minimal notification of their rights to file a claim. The Canadian government showed little interest in the controversy, an attitude that was reported in a Canadian newspaper: 'When Robins finally recalled their products in 1985, Ottawa didn't launch a major advertising campaign. It simply "endorsed" the company's ad campaign advising women to have the Shield removed' ('Dalkon: A contraceptive ...' 1988, B5). In other words, it was left up to the American media to notify the public.

Language differences presented another barrier for foreign claimants. For instance, French-speaking Canadians did not receive notification in their mother tongue, so many were not aware of these events until much later. Many non-Americans could not have known of their eligibility to file a claim until it was too late. However, in some cases they were given an extension, which seemed to show a willingness on the part of the legal system to assist women and others who had not yet filed claims.

Without American Home Products' acquisition of Robins, the reorganization plan would not have been completed. Some may argue that this would have been a good thing. However, an evaluation of the pros and cons of the process could not occur until approximately ten years later. Its successes would be based primarily on estimates of payments to the claimants. For others, success would mean how well the people who had been affected had moved on with their lives.

In North American society, compensation for a personal injury is often sought through monetary means. Injuries can result in visible or invisible outcomes. When an injury is not visible (such as scarring of the fallopian tubes), the anguish associated with it is hidden. This can have a twofold effect: unless the injured party speaks of his or her loss, even those closely associated with the person may not be aware of her or his sensitivity to specific emotional issues surrounding the injury. The injured party therefore may not receive recognition for the pain. When such injuries involve loss of fertility, the emotional scars may run deep and the reminders of the loss are present on a daily basis (T. Maynard, Infertility Awareness Association, interview, 1 December 1995). Furthermore, proving infertility from the use of a contraceptive device can be distressing. The litigation process involved is usually emotionally draining and another reminder of the loss. However, there can be a sense of vindication for the person receiving monetary compensation if litigation surrounding such lawsuits is successful for the injured parties or claimants. Hence, the person receives a hint of recognition. For most of the claimants, nothing will replace the ability to have a child.

Alternatively, the litigation process may drag on for decades, leaving injured parties frustrated and confused. Again, this process is a constant reminder of the injury; it also delays the day of recognition for the injured. Hence, waiting for closure adds to the human cost.

The rules surrounding American and Canadian individual lawsuits against a corporation differ. Bankruptcy rules and proceedings against American and Canadian corporations also differ. The details of these differences can be found in any legal text. In brief, Uwe Manski, president of the Canadian Insolvency Practitioners' Association explains, 'American law is lawyer-driven, it is very adversarial; ours is much more driven by the need to sort out the mess, not declare the winner' (Stewart 1995, 80).

Despite the differences between American and Canadian law, some members of the Canadian legal profession quickly jumped on the bandwagon with American lawyers. However, the complications in cross-border litigation and differing legal guidelines created immense frustration for them. As a result, Canadian lawyers often found themselves in the position of farming out client cases to American lawyers. In most cases, Canadian lawyers acted as the liaison with American lawyers.

This offered naïve claimants a psychological comfort of sorts – someone was looking after their case. Nevertheless, this occasionally meant higher contingency fees for the claimant.

The cross-border complications also caused chaos for those legally representing cross-border clients. American lawyers expressed bewilderment about the Canadian claimants' caution in dealing with them. In some cases, the claimants felt isolated from the legal battle despite legal assistance. At times, a sense of loneliness emerged as a result of the geographical distance between claimants and lawyers. Some lawyers communicated with their clients infrequently; others attempted to provide a comprehensive view of individual cases. In this sense, lawyers provided a service that became a 'necessary evil.' Ultimately, claimants had to give up a large portion of their awards to the lawyers as part of the agreed-upon fee.

Similarly, many judges who played a role in presiding over some of these cases displayed divergent attitudes. Some remained neutral in their decision-making, others displayed intolerance for the perceived disobedience of legal representatives, and others voiced their disgust with the attitudes of many of the corporate CEOs.

Prior to the appointment of Judge Robert Merhige, Jr, Judge Miles Lord (one of the many judges appointed to these cases) presided over the Robins case. Lord voiced his opinion firmly to CEOs of Robins: 'It is not enough to say, "I did not know," "It was not me" ... Time and time again, each of you has used this kind of argument in refusing [sic] to the world that the chief officers and the directors of your gigantic multinational corporation have no responsibility for the company's acts and omissions' (Perry and Dawson 1985, 207). Lord pleaded with the company to stop its 'monstrous mischief' and to recall the Dalkon Shield (Perry and Dawson 1985, 208). It was shortly after this adamant stance that Lord was mysteriously suspended and ultimately removed from the case: '[T]he [Robins] company asked the Eighth Circuit to disqualify Lord from presiding over the litigation' (Mintz 1985, 229). It was this kind of activity that often delayed the process, frazzled the lawyers, and motivated activist groups.

In June 1974, Dr Donald Christian published an article in the *American Journal Obstetrics Gynecology* on the dangers of the Dalkon Shield.

That same year the FDA rejected the recommendations of action against Robins and the Dalkon Shield. Despite this, Robins suspended the sale of the Shield for fear of future repercussions from the FDA, but the company did not inform women of the Shield's dangers. It was not until 1980 that a warning was issued by the FDA recommending that doctors remove the Shield from long-time users ('Miamian gets 4.9 million ...' 1983; S. Shainwald, interview, 4 December 1995; Sobol 1991). The details on the dangers of the Dalkon Shield were not formally brought to the attention of the medical community and to some of the patient community until 1985. It was only at this point that Robins announced a program to inform women to have the Dalkon Shield removed.

Across the border, a news release from Health and Welfare Canada announced that A.H. Robins Company of Canada Ltd., Montreal, had suspended distribution and sale of the IUD (HPB 1974). This same news release referred to a nationwide survey in relation to all IUDs at the time.

The Robins corporate leaders got off with minimal penalty. The company still exists behind the protective merger of American Home Products and the Chapter 11 bankruptcy code. Dr Hugh Davis died in October 1995. Prior to his death, he remained adamant that the Dalkon Shield was a safe contraceptive device. He also continued to believe that the accusations against him were based on a political and corporate conspiracy.

The fallout from these deeds is so widespread that it is difficult to imagine how far it may extend after the Dalkon Shield claimants have been paid off. The human costs will far outreach the monetary costs. For some, the direct injuries to women, their spouses, and their marriages will fade into the background. Others will remain haunted by the loss of what could have been in their future.

3

The Female Survivors

In May 1971 Nancy asked her doctor for a contraceptive that would allow her to delay having children until she and her husband were more financially secure. She and her husband wanted something more convenient than a barrier method, such as diaphragms or condoms. Since Nancy was allergic to oral contraceptives, another solution had to be found.

Nancy's family physician had recently returned from a U.S. contraceptive convention where she had picked up about twenty sample Dalkon Shield IUDs. 'The Dalkon Shield file card (actually a set of cards given in a small folder to doctors for future reference) promoted the Shield as "the modern sophisticated intrauterine device with superior ... rational design." It also claimed it prevented pregnancy "without undue side effects, such as menstrual cramping." It also purported to be "well suited for nulliparous as well as multiparous patients" and to have "exceptional patient tolerance."' (Perry and Dawson, 1985, 69).

On the recommendation of her doctor, Nancy had the Dalkon Shield inserted. She recounts the experience: 'When I had it put in I could hardly walk; it was painful going in and ultimately, painful coming out ... I remember crouching in the car ... when I went home I was not feeling good at all ... I was feeling bloated ... I finally phoned my doctor two days later!' Nancy's doctor told her to hang on, 'You are going to have discomfort because you have not had children; it will settle' (Nancy, interview, 14 October 1995).

Nancy struggled through the next month hesitant to call her doctor again. She had fifteen-day periods, endured unusually heavy bleeding, and became weaker and weaker. Intercourse was very painful for her and her husband. According to Nancy, her husband complained that the string scratched his penis during intercourse.

Finally, she couldn't stand the pain any longer; she went back to her doctor. Again, the doctor told her to give it time: 'It will settle down by the third month.' The pain was too much, yet Nancy hung on because she believed her doctor knew better. She also felt that she and her husband had to wait a little while longer before they could start their family. At the third or fourth month the IUD did settle and the pain subsided. Nancy's periods shortened and it seemed that everything had worked out for the best. This relief, however, was not to last.

In November 1971, Nancy had another flare-up comparable to the pain she had experienced when the IUD was first inserted. Angry and in pain she went to her doctor and demanded that the IUD be removed. 'I want it out now, I don't care, I want it out now!' The doctor examined her and informed Nancy that the IUD was embedded in her uterus. This meant she would have to go into hospital to have it surgically removed. The doctor's receptionist called Nancy shortly after with a hospital date for late February 1972. Nancy was infuriated; this meant another three months of painkillers. Again, she felt she had no alternative but to follow the doctor's recommendations.

On 3 February 1972 Nancy became very ill. While at work, her vision blurred and people appeared to be floating in front of her. She thought she had the flu. Nancy regained her balance and booked off sick for the rest of the day. While in the car she began vomiting, and continued to do so when she arrived home. She lay motionless at home on her bed. When her husband got home, he was alarmed by her greenish complexion. When he called the doctor she told him to buy and administer an enema. After the enema, Nancy's lower abdomen momentarily felt better, yet, she was still vomiting profusely. She recounts, 'It didn't hit me until later in the night when I awoke in a cold hot sweat ... my husband was still sleeping. All I wanted was cold, so I placed the side of my face against the toilet bowl, just to feel coolness. I remember looking in the bowl and thinking: "Oh my God, this is green!" ... Suddenly it clicked; it was poison, I had peritonitis!'

Nancy yelled for her husband. After a flurry of phone calls to the hospital she was rushed to the emergency ward, where she was immediately pumped with penicillin and painkillers. Three doctors surrounded her bedside. One doctor, a gynecologist, examined her and asked her if she had an IUD. Nancy replied, 'Yes, I know now that's what is causing this.' The doctor reached inside her, pulled the IUD out without hesitation, and asked, 'Who put this in you?' Later the doctor described the inside of her uterus as a 'smouldering forest fire that had become inflamed.'

Nancy told the gynecologist that her family physician had inserted the Shield. This physician never visited Nancy at the hospital, and Nancy never made another appointment with her again. She was disappointed that someone she had trusted had basically ignored her condition. Nancy stated, 'When I first had the Shield inserted I was about twenty and very shy, not very assertive ... that's why I chose a female doctor; I thought she would understand my needs better than a male doctor.' She quickly realized that gender is not necessarily a reliable criterion for a caring physician.

Nancy remained in the hospital for approximately three weeks still not believing what had happened to her. She kept asking her husband to bring her clothes to the hospital so they could attend a social function. He was bewildered and concerned. Between these requests and Nancy's denial of illness, she floated in and out of consciousness. She continued to be ill. Finally, the doctors informed her that she needed exploratory surgery. She could not believe it.

The day of the surgery arrived. Nancy says, 'One morning I awoke out of a dead sleep and a nurse was prepping me for surgery ... Two days later I awoke fearing they had taken everything.' They had wanted to perform a hysterectomy; fortunately, her husband had refused to sign the consent form. He still wanted them to have a chance to have children, and so did Nancy.

Afterwards, the surgeon informed her that infection had spread throughout her system and her insides looked like minced meat. The remaining scar from the surgery was a mess: Nancy's naval was pushed to one side and the bulk of her abdomen appeared lumpy.

Nancy's recovery took over a year. Weekly visits to the doctor and good care led to improved health. Nancy and her husband still remained hopeful that they would have children. In fact, they both were in their mid-twenties so it seemed the ideal time, but Nancy's doctor told her,

'You weren't expected to live ... Everything seems normal now, but it is unlikely that you will be able to conceive.' She was in denial and afraid to tell her husband. He was enraged and wanted to sue all the doctors. Then Nancy blamed herself. She had fertility tests that confirmed her physician's suspicions. Her husband insisted they adopt children. Nancy said, 'I wasn't ready to have someone else's child; I was still recovering from the news that I could not have my own!' She went to another doctor and told him her story. He referred her to a U.S. lawyer who was handling Dalkon Shield lawsuits.

Nancy's lawyer felt her case was strong enough to file a $5.6 million lawsuit. However, the litigation process was going through its own upheavals. Her case was shuffled from 1985 to 1987 and slotted in with the numerous other cases within the A.H. Robins bankruptcy plan. By now Nancy was devastated, emotionally fed up, and tired of people telling her what to do. She left her first husband in 1974: 'I only intended to take a three-week reprieve from the intensity of the last few years ... but I never went back ... suddenly being on my own allowed me room to heal!'

Eventually, Nancy and her ex-husband both remarried and moved on with their lives. For the next twelve years Nancy's life was relatively positive. She still had leakage and pain in her left groin, but this did not interfere with her daily functioning. In 1980 when she remarried she had cosmetic surgery on her abdomen to repair the mess created from the original emergency surgery done in 1972. In addition, she underwent minor surgery for dysplasia in which the doctor scrapped and removed the abnormal cells from her cervix. Relatively speaking, Nancy was doing well, considering her life-threatening infection of years before.

Twelve years passed from the time Nancy had the Dalkon Shield inserted. She and her second husband had a nice home, and they had agreed not to have children. Then, one morning, Nancy doubled over in excruciating pain. 'I knew there was something wrong. I went to the doctor the next morning for an ultrasound.' He said, 'I don't know how to tell you this ... You have a huge cyst growing on your left ovary.' She was hospitalized immediately, and was advised by her doctor to sign a consent form in the event a hysterectomy was needed. At this point Nancy was only thirty-eight; for her, the doctor's advice was like a final statement that she would never have children. Finally, she accepted the possibility that when she awoke from surgery her life would be changed forever.

When Nancy briefly awoke from surgery her husband was by her side. She asked him, 'What did they take?' He replied, 'They took everything.' Nancy says that her husband told her later, 'You woke up a day later after surgery to ask me that question ... When I told you what happened, you just dropped out cold on the pillow ... you were gone! I thought you had died; I shook you ... then you slept for another day ... I felt really bad!'

Later, Nancy's doctor told her that all of her organs had been glued together from the adhesions that had developed from the first surgery. He explained, 'Your bladder and kidneys were stuck in with everything else ... They had to call in a urologist ... We were afraid we would cut other organs ... This was touch and go ... we almost lost you!' During the surgery, events escalated to a point at which the surgeons could not wait for the urologist, and Nancy's bladder was punctured.

Nancy recalled, 'I never forget waking up; the pain was excruciating ... I yelled for the nurse ... She insisted I stand up and walk ... I yelled at her that something was wrong and to get the doctor.' The doctor arrived and assured her that the pain would subside in a few days; the pain this time was from the bladder surgery. Eventually, the pain did go away with cortisone shots administered to the pelvis. Also, Nancy's menopausal symptoms were balanced out with the hormone drug Premarin.

Between 1985 and 1987 Nancy had good health and seemed to be recovering well. She began working as a secretary for the surgeon who had performed her most recent surgery. Everything seemed to be going well. However, again this would not last.

One morning at work, she had another excruciating bout of pain in her left groin. After complaining to the doctor, he ordered an ultrasound test. The next day, he told her, 'I don't know how to tell you this; you have another ovarian cyst.' Nancy replied, 'How can that be ... you took everything out before!' He could not explain it until after the surgery, when he sat on the edge of her bed and, holding her hand, said, 'I don't want you to get mad at me, but when we looked inside and pulled the tissue forward there was a tiny ovarian tissue that had been left inside of you from the last surgery ... Somehow because of the mess inside, we missed it ... I'm sure you can understand.' Nancy recalled that the doctor was probably terrified that she was going to sue him. However, she sued A.H. Robins instead. She asked her first husband to support her efforts by writing a testimony to her lawyer about the sad events that he and Nancy had endured during 1972. He refused. Despite his remarriage, he remained bitter. Fortunately for Nancy, the hospital had kept her medical records that indicated she had had a Dalkon Shield.

Nancy refers to her last operation as a second hysterectomy. She had to go through the same procedure and recovery time as with the 'real' hysterectomy. Her doctor was equally upset with the results. Today, Nancy and her second husband live on the west coast of Canada and have moved on with their lives. In 1991 Nancy was awarded $148,000 in compensation. Her lawyer took 33 per cent as a contingency fee. Nancy has now released her lawyer and has also received another 85 per cent of her original award as part of the pro rata distribution from the Dalkon Shield Claimants Trust Fund. Although the money will never compensate her for her injuries, it does at least provide some recognition of the pain and suffering she endured.

Nancy's life is still not pain-free, but the pain is not as devastating as in previous years. It is only now that she has reached her forties that she is able to let go of the idea of motherhood. She says, 'I can only view these events in my life in such a way that I was not, for whatever reason, meant to have children.'

Many women suffered varying levels of injury from the Dalkon Shield. Some women incurred only mild infection and were able to have children. A relative few did not incur any problems from the Shield. For most, infertility was the tragic outcome. The women who experienced intense pain, numerous infections, near death, infertility, and broken marriages incurred the highest degree of human cost.

Scholars have examined the psychodynamics of these kinds of injuries (Anselmi 1994; Hicks 1994). The emotional trauma for the female patient survivors included anger, sadness, depression, and self-blame. Executive Director Trish Maynard of the Infertility Awareness Association in Ottawa, Canada, states, 'Infertility produces a great emotional impact ... The loss is like a death; it becomes a major life crisis for the person involved. There is a "bigger" anger when infertility is brought on by an IUD or what is called "physician error." There is a sense of lack of control and self-blame. Later, outward blame usually occurs ... The anger relates to a sense of betrayal' (T. Maynard, interview, 1 December 1995). For these women, it is not only a case of not being able to conceive; they are left with a feeling of having been violated by people who supposely knew what they were doing. Fifteen years after her experience with the Dalkon Shield, an injured woman expressed her anger at the manufacturer:

Physically I was very unhappy ... emotionally I was beat! I can just remember laying down, I was so damn tired ... no strength, and angry and hurting ... and then I started reading stories about women who had the Dalkon Shield – women who had never had children, and women who had children like myself and would have had another child, perhaps, and who had hysterectomies, and so on. And I thought this drug company was able to do whatever the hell it wanted, and nobody stopped it. It blew me away and then I got angry. Then I got really angry. (Anselmi 1994, 157)

A high percentage of the women who wrote about their experiences complained of the treatment they received from both male and female physicians. Poor treatment ranged from value judgments about the patient, such as suggestions that she was promiscuous or unclean. There was also frequent refusal to remove the Dalkon Shield along with a lack of general support from some physicians. This is evident by the frequent recollections of women who said that their doctor responded to their extreme pelvic pain and bleeding with statements like 'this is a typical response; go home and rest, it will go away.'

Although it is true that sexually transmitted diseases will increase the risk of PID, it is well documented that the wicking tail string of the Dalkon Shield was, in large measure, the culprit in this case (Tatum, 1975, 1976, 1977). The accusation that all women who used the Shield were promiscuous is preposterous. Numerous professionals in the medical field now concur that this suggestion was just another form of intimidation and blame from the Robins company.

Irene and her husband Gerry had been married since they were seventeen years old; they later had two children. For a variety of reasons they decided to delay another pregnancy, and Irene decided to use the Dalkon

Shield. To the couple's surprise, Irene still became pregnant. Her doctor recommended that she leave the Shield in place so as not to disturb the fetus. Five months into the pregnancy Irene experienced excruciating pain. Hours later she and her husband lost their son to an emergency abortion. As a result, Irene became despondent and moody. Gerry reflected, 'Irene's moods were so extreme that she was no longer the woman I had known for so many years ... We began to drift apart ... I didn't know what to do.' Irene threw herself into her piano. Gerry focused on his work and on raising their two teenaged children; his efforts kept the family together (Irene and Gerry, interview, 15 October 1995).

As Irene grew stronger, she became involved in Dalkon Shield Action Canada (DSAC) along with several other women. Much of her time and energy were spent in the activities of this group. Gerry then became depressed for a time. He had spoken with no one about his sense of loss over the son lost through a septic abortion. He did write, however, about his inner emotions to the lawyer who represented their case against A.H. Robins (Appendix B). Today, Irene and Gerry feel that their spiritual faith has helped them to heal from the trauma of losing their son.

Infertility caused by the Shield was a strain for many other marriages. Some broke up, others weathered the storm, and some became stronger as a result of the shared ordeal. Some married women did not have a supportive spouse throughout the ordeal. In these cases, many tended to blame themselves for this lack of support. For example, Sally viewed her husband's response as stoic, and made excuses for his absence: 'My husband is a stoic person, nothing ever goes wrong with him ... No I don't think he blames me for the Dalkon Shield, I think he somehow blames me for having the hysterectomy ... he was so angry that he didn't come to the hospital for 3 days ... You know he sounds like a shit, and at the time he was. It was just a crummy thing for him to do. He didn't know how to deal with it at this point ... he was so petulant ... He really didn't come to me at that time because he couldn't deal with it. ...We've resolved that' (Anselmi 1994, 153).

Often in cases of infertility it is couples that are given a high priority by the medical community and by society. Single women have another story. Barbara recalled her experience: 'After I told [my partner] I couldn't have children, no way possible, I never saw him again ... Even though I can't have children, I'm still a woman, I'm not worthless' (Anselmi 1994, 151). Sara also encountered rejections from men who could not accept her infertility. She recounts a conversation with a man that she had been dating for some time: '[He said] "I'm scared ... Because you can't have children ... I don't have kids." ... It hurt ... I mean it makes you feel like you're worthless, even though you know you're not ... Three men said that to me ... one I had been seeing for a year and a half. The last person that said it to me was the reason I said, "The Hell with [A.H. Robins]" And that's when I decided to find out more about [A.H. Robins injury claims] (Anselmi 1994, 151).

Other single women who became infertile as a result of using the Dalkon Shield have similar stories. They felt cheated as well as emotionally empty. One woman stated, 'It is difficult for people to understand ... Many can't relate to your experience because it is not visible. They don't imagine that you want children if you are single. The attitude is, well once you meet a man this will happen or you can adopt ... Well it doesn't always work that way ... Most men want offspring, therefore they want women who can have offspring with them ... your choices are limited ... it's as if you are on the sideline, alone.' (Mia, interview, 1995).

At the age of nineteen, Cathy Cameron was planning to travel to East Asia for the adventure of a lifetime. It was the early 1970s, and she felt there was lots of time to return to school. She was single and wanted a safe contraceptive to protect herself. She had a Dalkon Shield inserted a week or so before catching a plane to the first stop on her voyage, England. Cathy then intended to fly to Asia. She never made it.

Within a week of using the Dalkon Shield, Cathy doubled over in severe pain. She immediately went to the hospital, where she stayed for a week. Prior to removal of the IUD she was given heat treatment to help reduce the infection. The infection in her body forced her to remain in bed for approximately five months, but it was about a year before she was able to resume her working life. When she returned to Canada from England she contracted numerous infections, so her doctor placed her on antibiotics. An allergic reaction to penicillin caused her tongue to turn black and made her temporarily blind. Cathy recalled, 'My boyfriend was wonderfully supportive and dedicated to looking after me ... My

doctors were also very supportive ... In fact, the doctor in England provided documentation that stated the IUD was, in fact, a Dalkon Shield.'
Cathy says that she never had a burning desire to have children, so her
fertility was not an issue. However, her experience with the infection is
something she could have done without (C. Cameron, interview, 17 June
1995).

Women in underdeveloped countries tell of other horrors of infection,
manipulation, and death caused by the Dalkon Shield (Boston Women's
Health Book Collective 1994). Karen Hicks writes in her book (1994)
about these women who 'when injuries manifested ... faced both medical and personal dilemmas ... many of these women were intensely
anguished when they later discovered this device ... can precipitate an
abortion' (pp. 45–46). Only a small number of these women were even
aware that their gynecological problems stemmed from using the
Dalkon Shield. This was, in part, because information about the dangers
of the Shield had not reached many of them.

In 1972, Helena's doctor inserted the Dalkon Shield. 'He said it was the
greatest thing since sliced bread ... Little did I know that it would make
me infertile.' (Helena, correspondence and interview, 26 July 1995).
Later this same doctor was hesitant to provide Helena with a letter documenting the insertion of the Shield: 'He was terrified that I was going to
sue him; however, my lawyer assured the doctor he would be absolved
of any responsibility if he provided the proof of insertion.' The doctor
did eventually write a vague letter on Helena's behalf, but later
destroyed all of her files. Helena was saddened by her doctor's response
since she felt they had had a trusting patient/doctor relationship. Years
later, another doctor wrote her a letter confirming that her infertility was
definitely caused by the Dalkon Shield.
    Helena's first marriage was destroyed by the events surrounding her
use of the Dalkon Shield. Like many couples, she and her husband had
chosen to wait until their financial situation improved before having a
family. In 1977, they felt this time had come and were both looking forward to becoming parents.
    The couple tried to conceive for over a year, but without success.
'During that year my husband and I would break down in tears ... Many

of our friends were having children at the same time ... I wanted a child badly, I felt so inadequate ... I thought I was going crazy with frustration.' Helena became very discouraged.

In 1978, Helena's husband sank into a deep depression. He began having an affair with a woman who had three children. He eventually told Helena about the other woman, which caused her to panic. At one point, the other woman and her children would phone the house asking for Helena's husband. In an attempt to save her marriage, Helena suggested they both see their family physician. Their doctor encouraged her husband to have a sperm count done. However, he was not interested in doing this. The doctor then recommended that her husband seek psychiatric help to help with his depression. This attempt to help him was also unsuccessful.

Helena's husband left her for the other woman and remains there today. He seemed able to fulfil his desire for fatherhood as a stepfather. Helena was devastated for a few years. She says, 'If I had known that I would not be able to have children, I would not have tried to plan my life so perfectly.'

Life seemed hopeless for Helena until in 1983 she met an old friend who was also separated. They began dating, fell in love, and married in 1986. Helena cared about his two children, but she still wanted her own children. She went to a gynecologist to see if anything could be done to 'fix' her problem. She recalls that this experience was one of the most humiliating: 'His office was filthy and his bedside manner was deplorable ... He had a mobile hanging in his office made up of IUDs ... After he gave me an internal examination, he combed his hair while I still had my feet in the stirrups ... He made me feel cheap. The only good thing he did was refer me to an infertility clinic.' It was shortly after she met with an excellent doctor at the clinic that Helena learned that she definitely would never be able to have children. This same doctor provided her with the name of a lawyer in Baltimore who ultimately handled her claim against A.H. Robins.

Finally, Helena says emphatically, 'Not knowing anyone else that was going through what I was feeling, I found it very hard to express my feelings ... The Dalkon Shield took my choice away as to whether I wanted children ... No amount of money can ever compensate for taking away this choice.' As Trish Maynard of the Infertility Awareness Asso-

ciation points out, 'One of the things that infertility will do is take the
very best relationship and shake it at its roots ... Taking [a child] away is
like a disability, it really places you in a position where you have to
change those goals'(Laforet 1994).

Ivy Tremaine had bleeding and pain before she gave birth to her dead
daughter. 'This was the daughter I had always wanted; the priest bap-
tized her "Marie" before I had awakened from the childbirth ... That was
my Kim ... I had always wanted to call my daughter Kim ... They took
that away from me, too ... We don't count you know!' (I. Tremaine,
interview, 17 September 1995). Ivy had given birth in a small town in
Quebec where everyone knew one another. Her doctor was her first
cousin.

The doctor had advised Ivy to have the Dalkon Shield inserted shortly
after her first child was born. He boasted that the Shield was the miracle
of the century. Ivy had had the Shield in place for almost a year in 1972
when she became pregnant. When she informed her doctor of the pregnancy, he responded, 'That's impossible!' However, when he examined
her, he was obliged to confirm that she was, indeed, pregnant. He could
not locate the string of the Shield. At three months, Ivy almost miscarried, although the bleeding was finally controlled. It wasn't until she was
twenty-two and half weeks' pregnant that she felt herself losing the
baby. She recalls, 'I was afraid to sit on the floor because I thought, oh
no, this is it ... Finally I got the nerve to get up, then I began bleeding.'
Ivy immediately called her doctor. His response was to tell her to lie
down and put her feet up. It was not characteristic of Ivy to cry when
faced with discomfort; however, this time the pain was impossible to
withstand. She lay on the couch wondering when it would go away.
Later that night, she gave birth to her dead daughter.

Later Ivy had two healthy sons. However, the memory of the daughter she lost haunts her to this day and her anger towards A.H. Robins
persists. Ivy, like so many other women, lost her faith in the medical and
legal system, as well as her child.

Anne had the Dalkon Shield inserted for about six months when she was
twenty in the spring of 1973. During that time she developed severe PID
and spent two weeks in the hospital. Anne wanted children; two ectopic

pregnancies later brought frustration and agitation for her and her husband (Anne, correspondence, 1995).

Anne had never before experienced such excruciating pain as during the insertion of the Shield. A few months later she visited her doctor complaining of recurring pain. After examining Anne, the doctor informed her that either she had an infection or she was pregnant. She was thrilled with the prospect of being pregnant. However, she did not realize the implications of being pregnant while still wearing the Shield. Anne was not pregnant, but she did have the notorious infection that many women worldwide were developing while using the Shield. After a series of fertility tests and surgery, she was told by her doctor that she would not be able to conceive because of infection. She was devastated and outraged.

Her husband, on the other hand, could not understand Anne's intense emotion. For him it was not a matter of great importance: if they had children that was OK; otherwise, it was not a big issue for him. Anne recalled, 'I felt guilty for pushing him to be tested [for fertility]; the guilt grew and soon it caused a strain in our relationship.' Despite this, Anne seriously contemplated adoption. The more she considered it, the more she came to accept this as the best alternative. Again, she had to go through a series of what seemed like intrusive questions about her personal life. Nevertheless, she felt she had to follow the rules to get what she wanted. Once the couple passed through this process, they were offered a wonderful little girl.

Unfortunately, a few years later, the initial gap between Anne and her husband had not mended. As a result, they divorced and both remarried. Anne says emphatically, 'The enormity of the deception, the lack of responsibility and the total disregard for the women who were to use this product is simply overwhelming ... Someday I want my daughter to know what pain this product caused for so many women.'

One of the most horrific stories is recounted by Nora, a mother of two small children. While using the Dalkon Shield, Nora became pregnant. In her fifth month of pregnancy she felt horrible. She was exhausted and unable to look after her children. She complained to the doctor who advised her that she was likely depressed because her husband was unable to offer her support because of his long working hours. Nora was alone with her children of five years and six months old when she suddenly began to miscarry. 'I delivered in the bathroom ... The ambulance from the volunteers came ... while I was sitting on the toilet the physician was on the phone and he said get something to cut the cord. And he neglected to say and save the fetus, so it got flushed down the toilet ... That to me that's the part ... nightmares ... that's the part that gave me the most ... I had enough sense to baptize it but I never thought at the time that I should have gotten something and taken it with me ... I'm sorry [crying]' (Anselmi 1994, 191).

What is perplexing about Nora's story is that in the end she apologizes for not having thought to gather the fetus. In the middle of the madness she still blamed herself.

'Numerous conditions were imposed upon claimants, in particular poor women of color' (Hicks 1994, 37). In addition, 'Insurance companies were requiring [the women] to sign liens against eventual settlements ... the agencies used the enforced liens in an attempt to recover monies they paid for women's medical expenses related to their Shield injuries' (Hicks 1994, 37). Such tactics appalled both claimants and activists.

The litigation process was twofold in its contribution to the recovery of these women. First, in some respects it prolonged the agony of waiting for some recognition for a wrong done to them. Second, however, it provided a light at the end of a long dark tunnel. For many, the end of 1999 would bring resolution of a draining experience. Some will continue to try to change a system that needs reminding that human beings are affected by the impersonal decisions and actions of institutional bodies.

Getting involved in Dalkon Shield activist group helped some women to redirect their rage. Their goal was to gain recognition and justice for all women in their position. The groups' story exudes the phenomenal energy of women who were willing to risk being further violated emotionally and financially by large corporate and legal entities. Some met in person, others only through correspondence, the telephone or the media. They came together from diverse parts of the World and became a voice for many women.

4

The Battle for Recognition and Justice

In July 1988, a confirmation hearing was held on the A.H. Robins reorganization plan. The Dalkon Shield claimants were allowed to cast votes in favour of or against the plan; many of these votes were made by proxy by the claimaints' lawyers.

Karen Hicks, a Dalkon Shield activist, was informed that she would not be allowed to address the court during the hearing with objections to the A.H. Robins bankruptcy reorganization plan, as she had done in the past (Hicks 1994). The order came from Judge Merhige, but was delivered through Merhige's right-hand man, Mike Sheppard. Hicks defied the order and was subsequently ordered by the judge to sit down. When she refused to refrain from voicing her objections, the judge had the federal marshals remove her from the courtroom. A long silence descended as Hicks was escorted out. In response, the other claimants stormed out of the courtroom and met with a Richmond, Virginia, television crew on the courthouse steps to express their outrage over the silencing of claimants (Hicks 1994). For whatever reason, Judge Merhige chose not to charge Hicks with contempt of court.

Karen Hicks, founder of the Dalkon Shield Information Network (DSIN), had on several occasions organized similar protest gatherings. Her personal magnetism was such that she was able to generate energy among the women to take a stand against the injustice of the reorganization plan. On one other occasion, activists from the United States and Canada contemplated chaining themselves to the gate of A.H. Robins's headquarters (L. Hightower, interview, 31 January 1996). On the same day, many of the claimants wore white felt Dalkon Shield badges on their shoulders as a symbol of solidarity. This was also meant to attract the media, which at the time were equally intrigued and perplexed by the activitists.

Media coverage at these gatherings was extensive, but Hicks believed the media really did not grasp the situation. She and other activists spent hours on the telephone explaining the history of the litigation surrounding the Shield to members of the media. It became an exhausting process. Finally, Hicks and her group found it more practical to prepare press kits of background material on the Dalkon Shield saga.

Hicks's boundless energy had generated such widespread interest in fighting for the cause that DSIN groups eventually numbered approximately twenty chapters across the United States. One of the most driven DSIN leaders was Vera Davis, the Los Angeles coordinator. In particular, she initiated one of the largest outreach efforts through the press to African-American women between 1988 and 1989. As a result of this press release, Davis was bombarded with telephone calls from thousands of women.

The Los Angeles chapter of DSIN also organized a protest march at Harbor General Hospital in April 1990 for women trying to access copies of their medical records. As a result of this march, the hospital authorities made an effort to provide some records.

Although the media at times provided a rhetorical platform for activist groups, it also had its own agenda, according to Laura Jones of Dalkon Shield Action Canada (DSAC). Jones became frustrated with reporters who did not take the time to examine the facts and instead interjected their own interpretations in their final reports. She stated, 'I came to realize that the interviewers had their own agenda ... This was evident in the formulation of their questions ... They wanted specific responses ... Basically, I was not able to say what I wanted to say' (L. Jones, interview, 25 January 1996).

Similarly, Jones remarked that some lawyers did not comprehend the substance of the issues. She recalled one incident when she, together with a Canadian lawyer, was interviewed on a Vancouver radio talk show: 'I became enraged when the lawyer commented in a derogatory fashion that "Well these women are all in menopause anyway, so what does it matter that they have lost their fertility?" ... I couldn't believe

what I had heard ... I became enraged and took over the interview'
(L. Jones, interview, 5 September 1995). Later she admits that the lawyer seemed bewildered and somewhat oblivious to her reaction. It was
clear to Jones that the lawyer had no idea what he was talking about.
Despite numerous problems, most reporters and lawyers did assist in the
exchange of information, although some of these professionals were
more informed than others.

Author and journalist Morton Mintz of the *Washington Post* wrote
accurate and extensive articles on Dalkon Shield events. He had among
activists and some lawyers an impeccable reputation for detail and accuracy in his reporting. Mintz had also written an in-depth account of the
Dalkon Shield saga in his 1985 book *At Any Cost: Corporate Greed,
Women and the Dalkon Shield*. Mintz's accounts were based on reviews
of corporate memos, letters, and medical records, and interviews with
lawyers and top Robins administrative brass who were quite willing to
talk.

Lawyers such as Gary Thornton and Michael Leff of Atlanta, Georgia, supported the cause in part by financially assisting activist Linda
Hightower, founder of Dalkon Shield Victims (DSV), in her fight to
inform victims across the United States. Thornton and Leff picked up
the tab for her airfare and hotel rooms. This team effort involving several U.S. attorneys and Hightower aimed at ensuring that claimants had
some kind of legal representation and ample information about the
Shield. Hightower felt strongly that women needed legal representation
or advice before filing a claim: 'The legal and medical intricacies of the
Dalkon Shield were so complex that women really did not have a grasp
of what was involved ... and the Trust was not going to give them any
information, so they needed lawyers to represent them' (L. Hightower,
interview, 1 February 1996). Hightower herself formally released her
lawyer as counsel so there would be no conflict of interest. This also
meant that she would not have to pay a lawyer a contingency fee when
her case was settled. Instead, she requested advice from several lawyers
across the country. The lawyers, in turn, were provided with updated
information on the views and needs of many of the represented and
unrepresented women and men. For Hightower, aligning herself with
lawyers was the best way to help the injured.

Like many other activist leaders, Hightower dedicated her time and energy fully to help serve justice. She explained, 'We all had our own frustration and individual pain, we all found satisfaction in working with the other women ... but I was much more concerned ... that these women didn't understand the legal system or medical issues ... The other groups, I felt, were more interested in women's rights ... I was more interested in getting these women informed because they had such a big battle ahead of them ... Because I had another philosophy, they linked me with one attorney ... This created some unrest between myself and some other American activist leaders' (L. Hightower, interview, 23 October 1995, 1 February 1996). She was unique in her activist role in that she chose not to participate in protest marches. Instead, she preferred to gather information from court hearings to pass along to women who would call her for advice.

Because of extensive media reports, many women from diverse walks of life, and in some cases their spouses, joined in the protest against the Robins reorganization plan. Even if at the time they did not understand the intricacies of the plan, they did feel that A.H. Robins should be held accountable for its actions.

The increase in the number of women taking part in protest marches produced an image of a strong political collective. Such an image resulted in the women and their plight being taken more seriously by the media and the courts. It also encouraged other experienced activist groups to join in and offer valuable tips on successful activism and how to organize further media coverage.

Karen Hicks's early association with lawyer Sybil Shainwald provided Hicks with an inside track to some of the legal process linked to the Dalkon Shield. In part, this information became available to Hicks only through her persistent investigative skills. However, her persistence increased tenfold after she had joined Shainwald and author Susan Perry in an October 1985 talk show to promote Perry's 1985 book *Nightmare: Women and the Dalkon Shield*, co-written with Jim Dawson. This is when Hicks discovered the origin and scope of the tragedy (Hicks 1994). These new insights motivated Hicks between 1987 and 1990 to delve into the plight of all women who had used the Shield.

Sybil Shainwald was an avid health activist and successful lawyer. For Shainwald, health activism is her true calling; her legal work complements the other. Shainwald became an active supporter of Dalkon Shield claimants (S. Shainwald, interview, 30 January 30 1996). She was also a board member of the National Women's Health Network (NWHN), the Dalkon Shield Information Network (DSIN), and Health Interaction in the Netherlands. She registered many foreign women who otherwise would not have had an opportunity to file a claim. At times, Shainwald would meet American or Canadian claimants in distant countries such as Africa and direct them to people who would assist them with filing a claim. Her enthusiasm and drive comforted many of the foreign claimants. Shainwald remarks, 'No one else wanted foreign claimants with complex names; they didn't want to be bothered with complex spelling of the names ... Most American lawyers' attitudes were "Why should they (foreigners) get a piece of the pie?" ... It was disgusting.' She felt so strongly about this attitude that she refrained from working in association with a New York law firm because 'they were not interested in public interest work ... It was very difficult because after I started with them, they said they couldn't take care of those women' (S. Shainwald, interview, 29 January 1996). She immediately shifted some of her cases to a few lawyers who felt comfortable with foreign claims.

Shainwald paid her own travel expenses with the exception of one trip. The United Methodist Church paid her expenses to travel to Costa Rica in 1987. This was a fortunate trip for the women of Costa Rica, since most had not heard of the dangers of the Shield. Included in this group were nurses who also had not yet heard of the litigation. Because of the efforts of Sybil Shainwald and other activists, many international claimants became aware of their right to file a claim.

Those who gravitated to Shainwald often became leading advocates in assisting women with their fight for justice. These women called upon Shainwald for her expertise in the litigation process concerning the Dalkon Shield. In turn, Shainwald guided the women volunteers from a distance with legal or procedural advice with regard to filing claim forms.

Cathy Cameron, a Canadian claimant and activist, met Shainwald at a Nairobi, Kenya, health conference. Later, Cameron introduced Dolores Vader to Shainwald through a Dalkon Shield information session located at Women's Place, an offshoot of World Health Interaction in Ottawa. Shainwald instructed Vader on the correct procedures for filing a claim. In turn, Vader, who had a long history of working with the Vancouver Health Collective as a women's health counsellor, became the sole advocate in Ottawa for women who needed assistance with their claims.

Vader voluntarily worked eight hours a day counselling women, listening to their stories, and gathering medical records. She said, 'Many women would return from visits with their doctors and tell me that the doctors had refused to give them their medical records ... The doctors told them the records belonged in their hands and not the patients' ... I persistently told the women that the records belonged to them ... Women cried because of the sense of betrayal they felt from their doctors' (D. Vader, interview, 20 January 1996). The Canadian Medical Protective Association and the College of Physicians to this day insist that medical records do not belong to the patient but to the doctor. The patient is, however, entitled to a copy of her or his records.

Seattle activists Rosemary Menard-Sanford and Constance Miller formed the International Dalkon Shield Victims Educational Association (IDEA) in 1986. They spent hours attending to various inquiries from women and men about claim procedures. In total, IDEA accumulated approximately 2500 members from across the United States. The working nucleus was composed of eight to ten women, volunteers who were engaged in activities similar to those of other groups. They disseminated information to Dalkon Shield victims, advised women on legal matters, and appealed decisions of the courts. IDEA volunteers later aligned themselves with a Public Citizen Legal Advocacy group and met head-on with Trust officials.

Public Citizen Legal Advocacy lawyers Alan Morrison and Ralph Pittle, in particular, were of great help to IDEA in the pursuit of justice. Morrison and his colleagues were well-versed in product liability law, medical malpractice, and general legal counsel. 'Rosemary Menard-Sanford, president of IDEA, asked Michael Sheppard, the clerk of the bankruptcy court [at the time], for a list of names and addresses of all Dalkon Shield claimants so that a broader mailing could be conducted (Sobol 1991, 232). Sheppard refused the request, stating that Judge Merhige had asked him to keep the list confidential. Later, Alan Morrison filed a motion asking Merhige to instruct Sheppard to provide access to the list of names. A.H. Robins opposed the motion. Morrison and IDEA board members ultimately filed a petition with the United States Supreme Court to have the mailing list of claimants' names released to the public domain. After much haggling and many obstacles, the list was made available for a price (Sobol 1991). 'The list would help put forth relevant information about the Trust and court decisions to claimants internationally' (C. Miller, interview, 29 January 1996). Prior to the release of the names, activists such as Karen Hicks had to pay approximately sixty-five cents for each name they hand-copied.

Belita Cowan was founder of the National Women's Health Network (NWHN) and served as executive director from 1978 to 1983. In the early 1970s, Cowan's group received a package of material from an American midwest health collective about Mari Spehar, who experienced tragic repercussions from using the Dalkon Shield. Spehar's Shield perforated her uterus, leading to blood infection and her eventual death despite aggressive treatment with antibiotics. The midwest health collective came to be called the Mari Spehar Health Collective. Such extreme cases prompted Cowan to begin alerting Dalkon Shield users.

Belita Cowan's small network of women's health groups would grow to a national level by 1978. The NWHN then became one of the major players to petition the U.S. Food and Drug Administration to have the Dalkon Shield recalled from the market, although the 1983 petition was denied. The NWHN's main role continued to be a national health care information centre. It provided litigation services, a newsletter about current health issues, and general support for women who needed it.

Canadian activist groups were located in most provinces and several major cities. As with the American activist groups, the main goal was to share pertinent information with claimants and other activists. Cross-border communication between some groups was frequent, while for others the information flowed chiefly within their own localized area.

The Vancouver Health Collective, as with the Boston Women's Health Book Collective, had a mandate to provide, among other services, information, counselling, legal advice, and publication of general health issues. Trained volunteers, such as Laura Jones, managed the numerous telephone inquiries. Women telephoned in droves; with the innumerable calls about the Dalkon Shield, it became apparent to the Collective that a separate group would have to handle Shield cases.

Laura Jones and Elaine Cumley joined forces with Maggie Thompson and Megan Arundel and brought together other volunteers to create Dalkon Shield Action Canada (DSAC). DSAC networked with chapters of the organization in Montreal, Calgary, Winnipeg, and Toronto.

As time went on and the A.H. Robins reorganization plan evolved, divisive opinions emerged between some leaders. The differences of opinion were mainly about whether to align with lawyers or to depend solely on the decision-making of the Trust. Elaine Cumley, President of DSAC, campaigned aggressively for assistance from lawyers. She was insistent that women should get a fair deal. In part, Cumley's motivation stemmed from her own case, which had originally been filed early in the legal process, before the Robins motion for bankruptcy. Her injuries were so serious that her lawyer felt she could easily be awarded at least $5 million. However, because of Robins's motion for bankruptcy, Cumley's case, like many others, was set back on the list so that her number would not come up until 1987. This meant her case would be moved to an entirely different category and was now combined with the bulk of other Trust claims. The most Cumley could hope to be compensated was, perhaps, a couple of hundred thousand dollars.

Combined with her numerous infections, a hysterectomy at age twenty-five, and declining health, Cumley gradually began to weaken. The insult of being shoved down the list drained her emotionally and physically. Nevertheless, she continued her efforts to fight for justice by attending protest gatherings and conducting media interviews. She addressed the media despite ominous warnings: 'I was told a long time ago not to talk about this to the media or else I could have my case thrown out of court ... Women and families have been devastated and no one in the health system seems to be concerned ... If I lose my case, but save other women from pain, humiliation and devastation, it's worth it, because this sort of damage doesn't go away. The pain doesn't ever end' (Canadian Press 1987). Cumley continued the fight up to 1989, until she no longer had the physical stamina to continue. She died in 1990 from a brain tumour. Some members of DSAC speculate that her unrelenting pursuit of justice led to a breakdown of her immune system (DSAC, interview, 14 October 1995). Elaine Cumley died not knowing the outcome of her case.

Laura Jones, Executive Director of DSAC, advocated dealing directly with the Trust. She said, 'It didn't interest me, dealing with lawyers. We were connected with two other groups: Seattle and Pennsylvania (IDEA and DSIN). I thought we had enough information that we didn't need lawyers' (L. Jones, interview, 5 September 1995). It was at this point that tension developed between Jones and Cumley. However, it did not initially interfere with achieving their goal, which was to disseminate information to women and to lobby against the A.H. Robins reorganization plan.

Jones and Cumley valiantly pursued funding from a number of sources. They wrote members of Parliament for financial assistance, to no avail. At one point, they approached Health Canada in an attempt to get federal funding for their efforts, but this would not be forthcoming. Despite the lack of any substantial financial support, the activists continued to protest on behalf of the claimants. For the most part members of DSIN, as well as other Dalkon Shield activist groups, reached into their own pockets for expenditures. DSAC did, however, receive small donations from two lawyers based in Seattle and Vermont.

American and Canadian activist groups shared newsletters, information, and strategic plans for gathering lists of names of claimants. Numerous press conferences were arranged to reach as many women as possible. Most of the gatherings related to opposition to the Robins reorganization plan. Protests were held in Richmond, Virginia; Washington, DC; Seattle, Washington; and San Francisco, California.

In November 1987, six international women's health groups attended a press conference in Richmond that coincided with a three-day court hearing that was to estimate the total value of the Dalkon Shield claims. These groups included the International Health Network for Women, the Women's Global Network for Reproductive Rights, DSIN, DSAC, IDEA, and the National Women's Health Network. At the time, the A.H. Robins company was claiming a precarious financial situation. Thus, the focus of this conference became the fact that Robins was actually a very profitable company. Other press conferences and protests focused on the pending merger of Robins with another pharmaceutical company, the formation of a coalition in opposition to the plan, the rejection of the reorganization plan, and the firing of trustees (Hicks 1994).

In July 1988 Judge Merhige confirmed the A.H. Robins reorganization plan. 'The plan was approved by an overwhelming majority of Dalkon

Shield claimants. Of the total group of 197,000 Dalkon Shield claimants, 141,094 mailed their ballots back to the court. Of these 141,094 claimants, 94.5% voted in favor of the plan. Only 7,884 claimants voted against the plan. More than 99% of the 19 million Robins common stockholders who voted also approved the plan' (Hicks 1994, 69). Immediately after this announcement, lawyers and activists gathered in the courtroom to object to the decision. Both groups maintained that the Trust's promotion of the reorganization manipulated a high percentage of the claimants to vote in favour of it.

At the time, Elaine Cumley responded, 'This is very serious because a company was allowed to produce, manufacture and profit by a defective device ... if people are not made aware of the fact then it will be harder to prevent such a tragedy from occurring again' (Canadian Press 1988). In this same news report, Canadian lawyer Carey Linde stated, 'It's not justice ... the shareholders and the Robins family have made millions and millions of dollars. I believe criminal proceedings should have been laid against certain individuals involved with the Dalkon Shield.'

Some people were relieved that a decision had been made and the process could now move towards settlement for claimants, while others objected to what appeared to be a charade set up by the court system. Many activists felt that the legal process would not result in what the claimants had been led to believe would happen. No amount of protest would change Judge Merhige's final decision on the people's vote or revoke his final stamp of approval. For some, the defeat was overwhelming. They discontinued the battle and resumed the lives they had had prior to the Dalkon Shield litigation.

No one knew what the Trust was doing with the women's claim forms. As a result, an element of suspicion grew among many of the players. 'You never knew who was putting who up to what, and we knew the Trust had so much money and were so deviant that we were very concerned about who was an agent of who ... It turned out OK because we relied on one another to take up the call on various issues' (C. Miller, interview, 29 January 1996). Suspicion among activists and some lawyers escalated especially when the Trust seemed so reluctant to release any information about behind-the-scenes activities, projecting an atmosphere of secrecy and reserve.

Linda Hightower, who attended many of the lawyers' meetings, remarked, 'The blinds of all the windows at the Trust's location were always closed when you'd go to their offices. The Trust wouldn't let just anyone tour the building ... Why? Because they are paranoid, because they didn't want anyone to find out what they were doing, which makes you wonder what they are doing. Some attorneys considered going through their trash because [the Trust is] so secretive about everything, it makes you think ah ha! there's a lot here to hide. They justify it by saying it's all for the women' (L. Hightower, interview, 31 January 1996). In fact, if the plaintiffs' lawyers knew how the Trust handled the claims they may have been able to balance the process in their favour so that their clients would have done a lot better than the unrepresented claimants.

As a security measure, the employees of the Trust were instructed to exercise reserve when questioned by outsiders. One such employee of the Trust responded to a claimant's inquiry with 'Everything is a closed door, I can't tell you anything except what is allowed as public knowledge' (Anonymous Dalkon Shield Trust employee, interview, 15 December 1995).

Nevertheless, the task of helping the victims persisted. The Trustees now made attempts to ingratiate the activists by inviting them to Richmond to meet with them and Judge Merhige, tour the Trust's facilities, and discuss efficient ways to disseminate salient information to claimants. It seemed that the Trustees perceived the activists' networking skills and resources as invaluable. They also anticipated that they would now be bombarded with calls from claimants. A solution to this potential problem included, in part, working together with the activist groups. These groups were willing and able to handle this task, but their efforts would have to be voluntary.

The meeting in Richmond, if nothing else, would bring eight members of activist groups together. They would also get a closer look behind the scenes of the Trust. Some of the women met for the first time at this event.

Throughout this process, some of the activists and lawyers remained wary of the Trust's agenda. According to some, the Trust discouraged women from seeking the assistance of lawyers. Yet, lawyers urged claimants to avoid filing a claim against a multinational corporation without legal representation, which could seem overwhelming. Some claimants, at least, would need assistance of one kind or another.

For many women, filing a claim dredged up painful memories of the physical and emotional injury incurred from the Dalkon Shield. Many simply needed someone to listen to their stories. The Trust officers did not have the means to counsel claimants; they basically pushed paper and set policies. Lawyers as well did not have time to sit and listen to emotional accounts of injury. It only made sense that the Dalkon Shield groups and health collectives would provide this service. In some respects, the lawyers and the Trust needed the activist groups' energy and passion to assist these women. This volunteer work not only protected many women, but also provided a safe haven in which they could release very private emotions.

Many women needed to know the details of the culpability of the Robins company in the litigation process. Others needed help with filling out the twelve-page questionnaire designed by the Trust. Complicating matters was the fact that many of the injuries had taken place years before, so dates of events tended to become blurred. Clarification of dates then had to be found in medical records.

The complexity of the situation became overwhelming for many claimants. As a result, some withdrew entirely from filing a claim. Other women, who did not have medical records to prove the Shield had caused them injury, accepted the initial offer of a nominal award of $725. Constance Miller remarked, 'A letter from the Trust had gone out to the women regarding the funds with a suggestion that not enough funds would be available for the women ... the letter was trimmed in red and green [during the Christmas season] and offered women $725 ... Tens of thousands of women accepted this offer and then when their medical records showed up, they regretted it' (C. Miller, interview, 30 September 1995).

In the end, many activists did not feel satisfied with the results of the compensation plan. Many claimants would lose out; some would receive no compensation. As an example, the claim of one of the activist leaders took ten years to resolve. Ultimately, this woman, who had been rendered infertile, received an insulting compensation payment of $125. Several people who know of this case maintain that the woman's activism led officials to punish her for her advocacy work.

In contrast, other activists received figures in the $250,000 range. It remains a mystery to most why some cases were reviewed quickly and others were shelved for almost a decade. Those who had to wait more than a decade had filed prior to the Robins bankruptcy. A combination of events may have contributed to delays for many claimants. The reorganization plan, the frequent changes in Judge Merhige's decision-making policies, the shifting of cases from one lawyer to the next, the structure of the Trust administration, and the lack of substantive medical records may all have contributed to the waiting game.

As well, there seemed to be no acceptable explanation as to how the Trust arrived at a specific compensation figure. Some activists claim that a computer-generated point system devised by the Trustees determined the basis for the amount of the award (Hicks 1994). A Trust employee confirmed that, indeed, a computer-generated process combined with human decision-making assisted Trustees in arriving at specific offers for claimants (Anonymous Dalkon Shield Trust employee, interview, 15 December 1995).

However, some claimants stood their ground, refused the initial award, and went to Alternative Dispute Resolution (ADR), an appeal process that involves both sides negotiating a settlement with the help of a referee. Others who did not have sufficient evidence in their medical records also chose ADR. This allowed for an alternative to the options established by the Trustees. The awards for many of these claimants were increased by one to a few thousand dollars. Some were not raised at all. Ultimately, the credibility of the claimant combined with the bias and skill of the lawyers and referee at the hearing determined the monetary award.

For many claimants, the years of waiting for a settlement, the humiliation, the anger, and the legal expenses added insult to injury. They and their families found the entire process exhausting and just wanted to get on with their lives. Others wanted resolution and peace for themselves. Unfortunately, many faced several more years of waiting for this peace.

5

The Waiting Game

Jennifer Taaffe of Atlanta, Georgia, was twenty-three years old before her case could be heard at an Alternative Dispute Resolution hearing. She had waited since birth for recognition of her injuries. Jennifer was conceived when her mother was using a Dalkon Shield. The doctors advised her mother to leave the Shield in place to prevent injury to the child. Unfortunately, the Shield perforated the uterus. At Jennifer's birth, premature separation of the placenta caused her oxygen to be cut off. It was a tough delivery. Later, Jennifer's mother demanded that the Shield be extracted.

At birth, Jennifer weighed eight pounds (3.6 kg) and seemed healthy. As she got older and began school, however, she had increasing difficulty in identifying words. She saw some of the words backwards; at other times, she seemed to see words in sentences that were not there. Eventually, Jennifer was diagnosed with dyslexia. The prognosis was that she would always struggle with reading and writing.

In 1986, Jennifer and her mother both filed claims for injury caused from the Dalkon Shield. Seven years later, Jennifer was offered a settlement of $6,000. The news came as a blow: 'I was outraged. These people almost killed both my mother and me and they think that $6,000 is enough' (J. Taaffe, interview, 4 February 1996). She discussed the matter with her lawyer and they decided to reject the offer and shift the case to ADR. At least during this process, Jennifer would have an opportunity to voice her opinions at the hearing. A Trust lawyer, referee, and her lawyer would be present in the conference room. At the hearing, Jennifer expressed her disappointment with the original award offer and also provided an exhaustive account of her years growing up with a learning disability. The hearing went well and Jennifer was awarded the ADR capped figure of $20,000. The final report, in part, stated that 'evidence is clear in this case that Jennifer (nee Hightower) Taaffe experienced injury as a result of traumatic birth' (J. Taafe, interview, 4 February 1996). Her injuries included respiratory and neurological problems during birth, resulting in language and learning disabilities.

The Trust had twice changed the cap on ADR awards. Initially, in January 1993, the cap was set at $10,000; on 1 January 1994, it was increased to $20,000. Jennifer was fortunate in some ways that her ADR hearing came at the later date. Many women who took this route received the $10,000 cap. In effect, those whose cases fell within the earlier time range lost half of what they could have been awarded. Changing the rules was not an uncommon occurrence throughout the litigation process; many claimants and their lawyers were kept guessing as to when Judge Merhige would make another policy change.

Nancy Varney of Colorado was initially offered an award of $3,000 by the Trust. She was appalled at this lack of recognition for her injuries, which included long-term bleeding and multiple infections. Based upon the recommendation of her doctor, she also had an hysterectomy. Later, she discovered from her medical records that a hysterectomy had not been necessary.

Varney debated whether she had lost out by not accepting a lawyer's assistance. However, two lawyers had advised her that the details of her medical history were fairly straightforward and would permit her to defend her own case without risk. Prior to the final result of the hearing, Varney had waited more than ten years for confirmation that the Trust would help vindicate her losses. When she received their first offer, she was devastated and angry. She decided to appeal her case, which meant waiting a few more years before she could voice her opinion at the ADR hearing.

In preparation for this hearing, Varney examined her medical files extensively and researched medical terminology. Her in-depth examination of the details pertaining to her case was primarily intended to build a strong defence. However, along the way she discovered some disturbing errors in her medical files. The doctor's notes indicated that Varney's first husband had been found with discharge. In fact, the note should have read that he had been found dead (N. Varney, personal communication, 4 February 1996). Although Varney pointed out this error, the Trustee representative used this information against her claiming that Varney had contracted PID from her husband and not the Dalkon Shield. The referee's aloof behaviour, the Trust representatives apparent disregard for the facts, and the blatant devaluing of Varney's credibility disturbed her immensely. Her non-legal background had not prepared her for the cold and devious manner in which the process was carried out. The entire experience was a rude awakening for Varney.

For many claimants, the waiting game involved just waiting. Generally they were at arm's length from the litigation process and the Trust decisions and depended on their lawyers to explain what was going on. Sometimes the communication between lawyers and claimants was vague, giving many claimants the message 'I don't know any more than you do.'

Linda Hightower's case was delayed for many years. 'They [the Trust] could never give me a reason why it took so long. They just kept saying my case was tied to my daughter's and we had to be one case. That didn't make much sense' (L. Hightower, interview, 4 February 1996). By this time, Hightower's daughter Jennifer Taaffe was an adult and her case no longer needed to be linked with her mother's. After a six-month battle, the Trust agreed to separate the two cases.

For Hightower, the whole process of waiting for her and her daughter's claims to reach resolution was terribly frustrating. Her involvement with activism also added to the tension of waiting, primarily because of her awareness of the internal conflicts within the Trust's policy-making and the court's hearing activities. She said, 'I became so upset that I had to try to ignore it and pretend at times that it didn't exist in my life. I thought it would never end ... I thought I would be happy when I got my cheque. I didn't feel anything. I just felt numb ... it was like, oh there's a cheque; there was no sense of exultation or sense of closure' (L. Hightower, interview, 4 February 1996). Hightower felt cheated throughout the process, but didn't quite know where to direct this anger.

Lawyer Mike Pretl described the period between filing a claim and final resolution for one claimant as horrifying. This woman had filed a claim in 1982 before Robins filed for bankruptcy. Pretl frequently informed her that he expected to have her case settled within a short period of time, and he firmly believed this would be the case. However, delays within the court system and in organizing the Trust administration put many cases on hold. Some of these delays related to adjustments of the initial guidelines defined by Judge Merhige involving such matters as estimates of funds needed for the Trust, pro rata distribution, contingency fees for lawyers, firing of trustees, estimates of the Trust's budget, categorization of injuries, and so on. During the process of waiting to have her case heard the claimant went through personal bankruptcy to pay her child's medical bills. The child had been born with a brain tumour and died a few years later (M. Pretl, interview, 8 February 1996).

Judge Merhige's confidence in the payment process was sometimes unrealistic. Pretl recounts, 'I remember attending a meeting with Judge Merhige in 1985 when most women filed their claims. Merhige stated at that time that he felt assured that women would be paid by September 1986' (M. Pretl, interview, 8 February 1996). The reorganization plan, however, was not confirmed until July 1988. The administrative activities related to establishing the Trust and assigning work roles did not conclude until 1989. Pretl's client did not receive payment until 1992, at which time she had switched to a new lawyer who took a huge percentage of her $480,000 settlement as his fee.

Pretl decribes how the delay in compensation created other repercussions for many claimants. Some experienced marital problems as a result of the tension surrounding the situation. Others waited for a settlement before trying to adopt a child, only to find that they were turned down by adoption agencies because they were too old when they finally received compensations. The same thing happened to couples who waited for compensation before trying *in vitro* fertilization: in most regions, women under forty years of age are preferred candidates for this procedure.

For Laura Jones, as with many women, the waiting manifested itself long before the bankruptcy reorganization plan. She and her husband patiently tried for two years for her to become pregnant. Nothing happened. Tension in the relationship emerged. Worry and concern led her to have fertility tests. She was told she had damaged fallopian tubes. The news of her infertility left her and her husband devastated. Ultimately, they worked through their inability to have children together.

Mia filed a claim in 1986. Prior to 1995, she had been offered a $5,000 award. She was stunned and then angry, and turned it down. Upon the advice of her lawyer, she decided to challenge the decision. At the time of the first offer Mia was in her early thirties. While waiting for a new offer she went back to school in order to advance her education. 'In part, I didn't focus on the outcome because I was so busy. On the other hand, as a student, I could have used the award to help pay for tuition' (Mia, interview 8 February 1996). As for many claimants, Mia felt isolated from the litigation process by the geographical distances involved. She was enraged by her lawyer's lack of communication about delays or progress related to her case, and had to initiate calls at her expense to her lawyer about every six months. On one occasion, nine months had passed before she realized she had not heard from him. Mia had assumed that he was taking care of the details during this time, but he had not initiated any further action with her case. She was furious as well as by this 'Out of sight, out of mind' attitude. The lawyer told her that he had many other cases to attend to. The lawyer negotiated with her to have her case shifted to Alternative Dispute Resolution, and Mia agreed.

It was another year before Mia would be able to attend the ADR hearing in Philadelphia. Her lawyer did not attend the hearing; instead, the firm sent a junior lawyer to represent her case. During the hearing Mia was asked only a few brief questions about her case. Then the lawyers exchanged their evidence and chatted for a while about who knew whom in the legal profession. During the hearing, the Trust representative argued that Mia's medical records proved she had used a Dalkon Shield, and had had pelvic inflammatory disease, but there was no evidence that she had been treated for infection. This suggested a lack of sufficient evidence for monetary compensation. Mia quietly questioned her lawyer at this point. He urgently silenced her by gesturing that it did not matter. Mia insisted on providing a personal monologue of the human cost of her injuries. After the hearing she questioned the lawyer again. He responded, 'Oh that was up to the para-legal in our office to find that information.' She was infuriated at his *laissez-faire* attitude.

The final analysis of Mia's case indicated that she had presented herself as a credible witness. Mia believes that her passionate statement about the pain her injuries had created and her subsequent infertility convinced the arbitrator of her credibility. She was offered $12,000 in compensation.

Ivy Tremaine experienced some ridicule from her small Quebec community for filing a lawsuit: 'Some nurses where I worked made nasty comments about me filing a claim. I heard from a colleague that one of the nurses questioned why I had an IUD inserted, if I later wanted a child. At the same time the nurse suggested that I was just out to get money from the pharmaceutical company' (I. Tremaine, interview, 10 February 1996). Tremaine was furious and suggested the nurse read the medical literature and newspaper articles before making such ludicrous judgments. In part the comments motivated her to fight in the courts on behalf of all Quebec women. However, her battles in the courtroom left her saying, 'I wouldn't want to ever go through that again. It is exhausting. I've seen so many lawyers, it's sickening ... I've had it up to the eyeballs with all of this' (I. Tremaine, interview, 10 February 1996). Yet, some moments have been rewarding. A recent thank-you note from a young woman touched her heart and healed her battle wounds momentarily. She also received several thousand dollars in compensation for her own injuries.

For Helena, a Canadian, just filing a claim presented frustrations. She spent an estimated thirty-five hours writing about her injuries for the lawyers, yet they continued to request more and more information. At one point, they wanted a photograph of Helena and other personal information about her financial investments. 'You felt like you were being treated like a criminal ... it reflects a lot of women's concerns. No matter what it is, rape, domestic abuse, you feel like you have to prove your innocence' (Helena, interview, 10 February 1996).

Helena's frustration was compounded by the fact that she had a Canadian lawyer and an American lawyer. The Canadian lawyer was helpful in that Helena could initially discuss her case with him face to face, but later his communication with her became less frequent. She stated, 'I felt it was an up and down game ... They made it sound so positive and then six months later they would write a letter stating there would be delays ... They would build up your expectation and then like a roller coaster you'd be brought down again with negative news' (Helena, interview, 10 February 1996). Helena emphasized that her frustration was never about the money, but about wanting people to know the facts about the

Dalkon Shield story and wanting someone to take responsibility for the injuries she had suffered.

Some women were asked by their lawyers to complete a twelve-page questionnaire. Cathy Cameron stated, 'This long questionnaire was probing about one's private life. I felt a certain level of vulnerability. I also wondered if by answering some of the questions I was jeopardizing my case ... They also sent me a form asking me to sign over permission for the law firm to inquire about my financial records, professional career, and a few other things. Again, I felt very isolated in all of this and didn't know who to ask.' (C. Cameron, interview, 9 February 1996). Cameron sent the forms back to the lawyers incomplete, as did other women. They challenged the logic of answering such invasive questions; demanding to know how these related to their case. Cameron's lawyer never responded to her rejection of the questionnaire.

Some husbands left their wives as soon as they realized that they were unable to conceive. One such husband responded to hearing about his wife's infertility with: 'I'm out of here.' This same husband was quite prepared to file a claim for his own personal losses and in fact was well within his rights to do so. However, his wife was more concerned with the breakdown of their marriage. She also filed claim for physical and emotional injury.

The computerized point system established by the Trust to determine the extent of a woman's injury did not always place much credence on the breakdown of a marriage. Constance Miller recalled, 'There had to be problems in the relationship prior to the infertility problems from the Shield ... many women didn't want to accept this idea ... they would become very upset' (C. Miller, interview, 29 January 1996). Several women did dispute this view. Many reported that their marriages had been stable before the infertility issue arose. Interestingly, some of the ex-husbands would make a reappearance in the women's lives when they heard of the final monetary compensation awarded to the women.

In one case, a woman asked her husband to leave the house because of his lack of support. He was furious. The couple did separate, yet never divorced. Ten years later, the husband made a conciliatory approach to his former wife. At this point the waiting game had ended for each of them. He had received a $50,000 award for loss and suffering. She had received $70,000.

Barbara Di Mambro, MSW, who counselled some of the Dalkon Shield victims, explained that in some instances, women felt responsible and guilty about their use of the Shield. Others felt confused by the legal forms and process of a lawsuit. Others would not feel relief from suffering until the waiting period had passed. An award assured them that someone had confirmed the culpability of the pharmaceutical company.

Di Mambro also stated, 'Most women I counselled would just suffer in silence ... I discovered that depression was a natural consequence of many losses suffered from the infertility issue and the physical pain of many who acquired PID' (B. Di Mambro, interview, 11 September 1995). Some women became so depressed when faced with the realization that they would never have children that it affected their daily existence.

Several women reported that outsiders could not fathom the pain associated with the injuries. It was invisible damage. Hence, the anxiety of waiting for closure was often hidden from others because of the nature of the injury.

The distance for women and men overseas was compounded, in part, by the mere fact that oceans and seas separated them from their lawyers. Correspondence through the mail took twice, sometimes three times, longer than domestic mail.

Irish Catholics incurred delays, in part, due to their own hesitation to file a claim. Many of these women felt fear and shame connected to filing a claim. Most of these women had the Dalkon Shield inserted in England because of conservative Irish Catholic mores. Others had the Shield inserted at Irish clinics, where some of the Shields had been smuggled. As a result, medical records were difficult to locate (Hicks 1994). Likewise, claimants in Puerto Rico, Australia, Asia, and Africa also had similar frustrations with waiting.

Much of the waiting game can be attributed to the long, drawn-out process of the court and Trust procedures. In addition, because of the lack of communication with foreign claimants, many of them missed deadlines and had to be slotted into later dates. Court hearings and events surrounding the merger of A.H. Robins with American Home Products also impeded the progress of claims. Many of these claims were delayed because of lengthy decision-making.

It had been anticipated by many lawyers that the completion of payment to claimants would take approximately two decades. In fact, closure of the Trust fund would likely not occur until 1999. Trial cases may extend into the year 2000, however.

Did the expediency of settling claims through the Trust compromise the fairness of the monetary compensation for claimants, or was this approach the best for the majority of claimants? The answer to this may lie in U.S. government records. Specifically, numerous documents associated with the confiscation of memos, records, and medical documentation on the Shield are with the FDA Department of Health and Human Services. The documents are accessible to anyone under the Freedom of Information Act. However, correspondence from the FDA office indicates that 'material has been deleted from the record(s) ... because a preliminary review of the records indicated that the deleted information is not required to be publicly disclosed' (M.T. Pivero, FDA correspondence, 29 January 1996).

The public will probably never fully know what went on behind closed doors. Some of the answers lie with those who participated in the legal process. One must wonder if they will ever feel confident enough to speak out publicly.

6
Lawyers and Litigation

According to some activists, the Dalkon Shield lawyers presented one or another image: the white hats or the black hats. 'DSIN leaders used a single criterion to define a lawyer as a white hat: that lawyer demonstrated a primary interest in the issues of justice and basic fairness involved in this case, not a simple focus on compensation' (Hicks 1994, 100). In contrast, DSIN leaders 'became increasingly uncomfortable and even angry with those ... thought to be motivated solely by their own aggrandizement' (Hicks 1994, 101).

As one Baltimore lawyer maintained, 'I think all of the lawyers manifested varied attitudes and behaviors in this whole process. You know, they all had to make a living; so, money had to play a factor in their approach to attracting claimants. But, I'd say many of the lawyers I knew also empathized with their clients' sorrow' (M. Pretl, interview, 27 October 1995).

Although lawyers were divided with respect to the appropriateness of the Robins bankruptcy plan and some of their colleagues' professional ethics, they were unanimously frustrated with the Dalkon Shield litigation process.

Lawyers were frustrated with the constant changes in the rules of the court and decisions made by the Trustees. The decision-making policies implemented by Judge Merhige enraged many. Some feared Merhige's iron hand; opinionated lawyers were threatened with being held in contempt of court or, worse, eliminated from representing further Dalkon Shield cases.

Other lawyers perceived Michael Sheppard, Executive Director of the Dalkon Shield Claimants Trust, as the worst possible example of an inflexible bureaucrat. Lawyer and author Richard Sobol pointed out that 'Sheppard shared with Judge Merhige the penchant for telling welfare-lady-in-the-Cadillac stories – such as the oft-repeated tale of a claimant who supposedly said she had taken two Dalkon Shields a day ... Sheppard was [then considered] an unlikely choice for the position' (Sobol 1991, 212). Apparently Sheppard and Merhige believed some women viewed the Dalkon Shield Trust as an easy 'get rich quick' scheme.

The Robins reorganization plan also outraged many of the lawyers. Some lawyers felt that the $2.45 billion in the Trust Fund would never cover the numerous claims and would once again leave the claimants in the position of victims. Some lawyers advocated a figure closer to $8 billion dollars, which would provide claimants, not to mention lawyers, with larger awards. Others felt that the Robins reorganization plan would at least provide monetary awards to a larger number of claimants. However, since these awards would be smaller, lawyers would have to take on more clients in order to make more money.

Some lawyers complained that claimants awaiting trial would be denied the same opportunity as those who had been awarded compensation prior to the Robins bankruptcy. After the bankruptcy approval, there seemed to be discrepancies in the awards. Lawyer John Baker said, 'I saw some inconsistency with two cases that appeared to me to be very similar. One was offered $35,000 and the other was offered $135,000, which didn't make sense ... I think we were three months away from going to trial on three cases. Because of the bankruptcy, those trials got stayed and those women never got to go to trial despite the fact that we had fully prepared those cases. We had forty such cases that we had been working up for trial and actually had done craftsmen-like work on' (J. Baker, interview, 15 November 1995). Not only did this imbalance infringe upon the rights of the victims, but it also would markedly decrease the lawyers' monetary return on such cases.

The reorganization plan also meant a ten-year delay that would ironically push some lawyers close to bankruptcy themselves. As lawyer Mike Pretl puts it, 'People talk about greedy lawyers all the time, and, yes, there are a lot of lawyers who have made a lot of money out of this, but essentially, lawyers subsidized clients' claims for the whole period of the bankruptcy' (M. Pretl, interview, 27 October 1995). In some cases, lawyers who did not have a strong financial base had to borrow $2 to $3 million from the banks to keep their heads above water. The fees they collected later went to pay off these loans. Canadian lawyer Christopher Kay confirmed, 'You cannot imagine the financial strain that this put me and my practice under. If it weren't for the bank having complete confidence in what I was doing I simply couldn't have done it. It was unbelievable how much debt I was in with this Dalkon Shield process. If it had collapsed, it would have wiped me out because my debt with the bank was enormous' (C. Kay, interview, 23 January 1995).

As a result of the smaller awards to claimants and the long waiting period, the contingency fees that some lawyers charged their clients for services rendered were way out of line. Fees of 50 and 60 per cent of compensation awarded to the claimants were at the high end of the scale. The average contingency fee was $33\frac{1}{3}$ per cent; other lawyers charged 25 per cent. Some lawyers, such as Sybil Shainwald, waived the fee for photocopying and postage on occasion for some claimants who did not receive a meaningful offer from the Trust.

Some lawyers justified their fees on the basis that claimants would have had to pay much larger fees if they paid lawyers an hourly rate. Nevertheless, there was some disgust with colleagues who charged exorbitant fees: 'Douglas Bragg and Bradley Post ... confronted other lawyers about the ethically controversial "wholesaling" and brokering of cases' (Hicks 1994, 100). Lawyers were also livid over Judge Merhige's decision on 1 March 1995 to limit the pro rata distribution contingency fees to 10 per cent instead of allowing the lawyers to collect the contingency fees they had already set individually. This was a major bone of contention for lawyers who had initially charged their clients a low percentage of the settlement offer. Other lawyers protested that they deserved more for their efforts in representing cases that brought in little return on the initial claim settlements, some of which were Option 1 cases. As lawyer Michael Leff put it:

We were fair all along with our clients and we got penalized the same as those who were not fair. Those of us who charged 25 to 30 per cent intended for that to be applied against whatever we obtained for the client – in one payment or more. Overall, we would come out pretty good. Under this present 10 per cent ruling, it isn't going to happen that way. If the claimants are going to almost double their initial settlement through these supplemental payments (which is now almost a certainty), then 25 to 30 per cent on the first half and 10 per cent on the second half, we are made to accept about 18 to 20 per cent overall. There was a huge risk in this for us in time and money and we bargained fairly with our clients. Once that agreement was made, it does not strike me as fair to interfere with our right to contract and to cut our fee in half. And it would not be normal for an attorney to accept a contingency case on 20 per cent. (M. Leff, interview, 17 December 1995)

On the other hand, other lawyers felt that a limit of 10 per cent at this stage of the process was adequate, believing that they had made a substantial return on many of their cases. Their thinking aligned with that of many activists and claimants who believed that 10 per cent was enough payment for writing a letter and a cheque.

Lawyer John Baker stated, 'Most people are going to be getting this pro rata distribution and I think it's very appropriate that lawyers only get 10 per cent. Even if the judge had not reduced it, I probably would have charged 10 per cent anyway' (J. Baker, interview, 15 November 1995).

Many lawyers did put their lives on hold to represent Dalkon Shield claimants. They had to educate themselves about the mechanics and impact of IUD contraceptives as well as gynecological complexities. Many hired nurses or doctors to assist them in interpreting claimants' medical files.

Some lawyers developed close ties with their clients. They knew about a client's personal hurts, dreams, and anger. These lawyers genuinely cared about their clients' lives as they learned more about their personal losses. As lawyer Christopher Kay put it, 'You know, you do this because you have a need to help adjust the balance in society ... so you get involved with these people, you accept them as clients and then basically as soon as you pick up the ball you're in there for the long run' (C. Kaye, interview, 23 January 1996). Likewise, some of the lawyers felt so strongly about the emotional impact on their clients that they have gone on to battle for breast implant claimants. Lawyer Carey Linde states, 'There was a sense of satisfaction in having been involved at least a little bit in "helping the small guy," which in this case was women, and, through the system, beating these multinationals' (C. Linde, interview, 12 September 1995).

Without a doubt, however, there were lawyers who recruited claimants with a vengeance. They travelled across North America and overseas as far as East Asia, Africa, and Australia. Some members of the legal community frowned on those who used blatant marketing approaches to recruit domestic and foreign claimants.

The polarized view within the legal community with regard to the behaviour and attitude of some lawyers also extended to the Trust administration. Lawyer Mike Pretl stated that 'Merhige did a masterful job of ramrodding this through; I still maintain that he got a great result. He stepped on everybody's rights including my clients', but he got a result of $2.45 billion, which frankly was beyond the wildest expectations of the victims' (M. Pretl, interview, 18 December 1995).

Merhige had a reputation among some in Richmond, Virginia, for being very non-judicial. 'What he would do is invite the lawyers around to his house for cocktails and sort of twist their arm to settle a large case ... but he does it very even-handedly. Most lawyers liked the guy because he has never been accused of corruption or of being unfair or biased. If he has a bias, it's in favor of the underdog' (M. Pretl, interview, 27 October 1995). However, it was not always apparent to all lawyers that Merhige favoured the underdog.

One lawyer recalled that Judge Merhige had initially praised the Robins family as being upstanding and important citizens who contributed to the Richmond symphony and other community activities. At the time, Judge Merhige suggested to claimants' lawyers in open court that they had the burden of proving to him that the Robins company was as corrupt as they were saying. Six months later, according to Mike Pretl, Merhige told the same lawyers that they had convinced him that some of the things Robins had done were outrageous: 'Judge Merhige now stated that he wanted to make sure that all of the money went to pay the victims' (M. Pretl, interview, 27 October 1995).

Judge Merhige was perceived by some as approving almost anything the Trustees proposed. On the other hand, many lawyers were concerned that he would slap the wrist of any lawyer or Trustee who spoke out of turn. As a Cleveland lawyer confided, 'A good portion of the docket – pre-bankruptcy materials, the trial materials, the discovery materials, the dispositions, video tapes, everything during the bankruptcy – is here, but we can't talk about it, that's the problem' (Anonymous Cleveland lawyer, interview, 18 December 1995). This statement illustrates the nervousness that some lawyers felt in exposing to outsiders certain elements of the litigation surrounding the Dalkon Shield.

Several lawyers expressed fear about speaking out against Judge Merhige or the Trust activities. Specifically, they were afraid that if they ventured to express an opinion about the litigation process that the repercussions would negatively affect their professional careers and their clients' cases. Others felt that there was no reason to be afraid as long as one spoke the truth. Sybil Shainwald explained it this way: 'My own relations with the Trust have been cordial. I don't have a problem with the Trust. I do have a problem with the amounts they awarded. For example, I think they should have had a higher limit on the ADR process because I think $20,000 dollars was too low. I also think we should have had a choice of mediators ... I have not said anything that isn't true, have I?' (S. Shainwald, interview, 4 December 1995).

The element of secrecy that surrounded Trust activities made many of the lawyers feel shut out of the process. More often than not they were not informed of changes implemented by the Trustees or Judge Merhige until the very last moment. This secrecy extended to many diverse areas of the Trust process.

Dealing with the multifaceted aspects of representing clients in a worldwide lawsuit against an American pharmaceutical company was stressful for everyone. For many of the lawyers, the stress affected their business, their family lives, their values, and their perceptions of their colleagues. As Michael Leff stated, 'There was no way to avoid the emotional involvement of understanding what these people had been through. I am at an age where I have a wife and a family that could have been subject to the same thing ... Now that I know the horrors that were wreaked upon some of the people, I believe they truly were victims' (M. Leff, interview, 27 September 1995).

Unfortunately, it was apparent that some lawyers were simply money hungry. Since the claims that provided the strongest medical evidence received the most attention and were most likely to provide the highest return, some lawyers actually weeded out the claims less likely to receive large awards. They either filed the less attractive claims under Option 1, where a flat award of $725 was offered to the claimants, or passed them along to another lawyer who willingly took them. Claimants who rejected Option 2 offers, ranging between $125 to $5,000, usually moved into the Option 3 category or chose to go to Alternative Dispute Resolution (ADR). As mentioned before, Option 3 claims often provided a satisfying result for the claimant and the lawyer. 'About 85 per cent or 90 per cent of the Option 3 claims have been resolved for the Trust offer. About 50,000 of 200,000 cases fell under the Option 3 category' (M. Pretl, interview, 18 December 1995). Canadian lawyer Carey Linde explains, 'As I got further into it I could see the real trickiness of it. If you were within Option 1, 2, or 3, you could answer just one question with a wrong slant and you could be pushed back from Option 2 to Option 1 ... If there were any injustices, it was the way the questionnaire was phrased and the way the medical consultants put it together. It was tricky. I came around to believing that if anyone even had a moderate claim they should have a lawyer' (C. Linde, interview, 12 September 1995).

A detailed account of a claimant's infection and subsequent injuries had to be recorded on her medical file by her primary physician in order for the Trust to give the injury serious consideration. The Trust wanted the straight facts from the physician who had inserted and extracted the Shield and subsequently treated the claimant. Hence, a letter from a physician summarizing a claimant's medical records did not suffice as concrete evidence of injury, according to several accounts provided by lawyers. This frustrated lawyers and, at times, impeded the progress of the claim process. Lawyer Mike Pretl said, 'The major beef I have with the Trust, and I have communicated this to Mr. Sheppard, is that they required contemporaneous medical documentation of everything. In other words, if I have a doctor today write a letter saying that Mrs. So and So's injuries, given her history, indicate she was injured from the Dalkon Shield, the Trust will disregard that unless I have the records from the time of injury ... In these cases the Trust will often offer them nothing ... However, this is a relatively small percentage of the claims' (M. Pretl, interview, 27 October 1995). Several lawyers interviewed for this book concurred with this view.

Interestingly, prior to the bankruptcy and with the onset of the ADR option, many cases were settled based on a woman's personal testimony of the alleged injury from the Shield. Nevertheless, lawyers stated that although the Trust produced viable results it often expressed scepticism about claimants' personal testimonies. The Trust also, according to some lawyers, usually assumed that claimants and lawyers were lying about the injuries in order to make money. It was commonly believed that the Trust too readily accepted the physician's word over that of the claimant.

Some lawyers either reduced their caseload or stopped representing further claims with the introduction of the bankruptcy reorganization plan. The complexities and bureaucracy of the bankruptcy process led them to direct their energies elsewhere. In contrast, there were those lawyers who remained faithful as well as opposed to the reorganization plan. On occasion, a claimant would reject the Trust's offer and opt to go to trial. More often than not these claims provided the largest returns for the claimant and the lawyer. Occasionally, however, the outcome of a trial and jury process was disappointing for the claimant and the lawyer. It was a risk that still, more often than not, paid off in a sense of vindication for both parties.

Those claimants who diligently filed earlier claims and those who accepted $1,000 or less discovered that they had opted for a one-time award. This meant that they would not be eligible for the pro rata distribution of funds. In contrast, those who filed at a later date with the Trust could receive the distribution of surplus money left over after the bulk of claims had been paid to claimants. For these very reasons, claimants and lawyers alike grew increasingly frustrated with the overall litigation process.

The settlement conference for many lawyers was an absolute waste of time. This process was meant to provide a platform for negotiation for those dissatisfied with Option 3 offers from the Trust. However, once there, the lawyer and claimant were not permitted to negotiate. Instead, they had to sit and listen to an arbitrator set out the facts of why the claimant's case was not worth a higher offer. The claimant often left the conference crying and the lawyer would leave infuriated. Both claimant and lawyer usually ended up going to court to dispute the offer. Unfortunately, some of these claims, after going through a jury, were not only denied an increase, but also the original offer was cancelled based on supposed new evidence discovered by the jury. Thus, the process was a high-risk one for claimants.

Lawyers from Canada were dependent on American lawyers' expertise. In some respects, Canadian lawyers' involvement with the Dalkon Shield cases straddled the Canada/United States border. In part, they became dependent on American lawyers and the Trust for relevant information about the Dalkon Shield judicial proceedings. This dependence resulted in a strong rapport between some of the lawyers on both sides of the border. Clearly, many of the American lawyers had the advantage in that they were familiar with the American judicial system. Still, both sets of lawyers seemed to have an understanding of the position of the other; they worked as a team by exchanging pertinent information. Consequently, Canadian lawyers often played the role of liaison with an American lawyer. They collected the cases and passed them along to an American lawyer who then processed the claim on behalf of the Canadian claimant. The Canadian and American lawyers shared the contingency fee. In some respects, the involvement of a Canadian and an American lawyer was useful because it added a sense of security for the Canadian lawyer and claimant. On the other hand, some claimants wondered: did they really need two lawyers to process their claim?

Some claimants and lawyers alike agreed that a lawyer was needed because of some of the complexities in filing a claim. For instance, Quebec women needed legal representation because of the absence of French correspondence from the United States. Many Quebec women had not been notified in French that they could file a claim in 1986. They were able to file late claims in June 1995 as a result of the efforts of Quebec lawyer Gratien Duchesne and activist Ivy Tremaine.

Duchesne filed a class action against A.H. Robins on behalf of Quebec women who were injured by the use of the Dalkon Shield. As he stated, 'It was the beginning of a crusade against A.H. Robins company which led us to the Supreme Court of Canada ... The negotiations with the Dalkon Shield Claimants Trust's attorneys took many years to result in the Quebec class action ... during those years I became aware of the bad consequences of the Dalkon Shield usage ... Without the class action more than 1200 people would not have been compensated by the Dalkon Shield Claimants Trust' (G. Duchesne, correspondence, 2 October 1995).

Physicians in every country involved were often initially uncooperative when asked to provide a patient's file or a letter to support the cause of the patient's injuries. There were several reasons behind this reluctance. Some doctors had simply destroyed the patient's file some years earlier, others feared being sued for malpractice, and still others simply did not want to bother looking for files that had been stored away a decade earlier. Canadian lawyer Carey Linde said, 'Most doctors were OK and eager to help, but the records in most instances in British Columbia were unavailable because policy said they only had to keep their records for seven years. Hospitals were completely obstructive by and large. Hospitals made you go through the worst ordeal. You had to get forms, pay outrageous amounts of money to get photocopies and they didn't want to be bothered with looking for them. But they did come around after the fourth, fifth or tenth time. They didn't understand what it was all about' (C. Linde, interview, 12 September 1995).

Often lawyers sought a claimant's medical records in part because of the slight chance that an X-ray taken for an unrelated injury might display an image of the Dalkon Shield. If such an X-ray was found, it meant concrete evidence was available to defend a woman's injuries. Generally, a lawyer wouldn't pursue such a lengthy search if other evidence showed indisputable evidence. Women also had to have medical records to prove that nothing else had caused their injuries.

Sybil Shainwald to this day adamantly maintains, 'To me, [Robins] was so wrong and did so much harm that they deserved to be put right out of business ... I think many women, if you ask them, "What do you want out of this?" they would have said, "I want the corporation to be punished."' Likewise, Shainwald blames the FDA for its lax regulations of the time: 'In 1974 and 1977 people went to the FDA and said, "Take this off the market." They didn't do anything. Every woman that was injured from that time on, I blame on the FDA' (S. Shainwald, interview, 4 December 1995).

Lawyer Robert Montague says, 'I think, historically speaking, there has always been a problem measuring damages to be awarded for emotional suffering ... there is always a problem putting a dollar value to emotional injury. If this had taken place in Canada, the maximum you could get, even in the worst case, is about $250,000 even for injuries resulting in quadriplegia. For pain and suffering there is a restriction. Yet, you could receive damages for future care, and future loss of income. That is where you get into the millions' (R. Montague, interview, 21 August 1995). Montague went on to say that in Canada this process would have taken a much shorter time.

After all is said and done, a number of lawyers who initially had grave reservations about the Robins bankruptcy and reorganization plan have decided that they were wrong. Many now feel that the overall process of awarding monetary compensation to just under 200,000 claimants was extremely successful. Michael Sheppard, Executive Director of the Dalkon Shield Claimants Trust, states, 'The people who did not get large offers are pretty unhappy. A lot of those people for instance ... we've had about forty lawsuits at this point ... have been very unsuccessful in doing any better than what the Trust offered' (M. Sheppard, interview, 14 February 1996).

Some Dalkon Shield claimants have received a final settlement offer and will continue to receive an additional pro rata distribution of excess funds based on their original claim value. Sheppard maintains that those claims that were timely, as well as late claims, received offers by the end of February 1996. Those choosing Alternative Dispute Resolution, arbitration, or trial will likely take longer.

The contrasting amounts of the settlements can seem puzzling; however, the average outcome has ranged between $30,000 and $35,000 for Option 3 nonrepresented and represented claimants. These amounts increased with the added excess funds. So, in effect, the eventual estimated monetary compensation for these people will amount to $60,000 or $70,000.

Many of the claimants not represented by a lawyer were offered $32,000. Interestingly, claimants who were represented by a lawyer received an average payment of $30,000 to $35,000 dollars. However, these claims were reduced when lawyer's fees were deducted.

According to Michael Sheppard, flaws in the system unfortunately led to attempted fraud. Those who provided false information or, in some extreme cases, false medical records, ended up with nothing. More often than not falsified records were identified and dealt with accordingly. For example, 'We basically kept the evaluation process confidential ... but [the claimants] can manipulate the records ... In fact, we had quite organized fraud attempts in the Philippines, which included falsifying of claims, false records, falsifying of individuals who were supposedly alive and really weren't ... We had various investigations and made a presentation to the court. Forty thousand of those claims were disallowed' (M. Sheppard, interview, 14 February 1996). Many of these cases had been falsified by a Philippine lawyer, but penalizing this lawyer was out of U.S. jurisdiction. The evidence of fraud was turned over to the Philippine police, but in the long run, fraud prolonged the waiting period for innocent claimants who had already waited years for compensation.

Sheppard's role as Executive Director of the Dalkon Shield Claimants Trust was not easy. His task was to make sure that close to $3 billion was fairly distributed to hundreds of thousands of people who filed claims with the Trust. In retrospect, Sheppard is able to view the positive and the negative aspects of the process: 'It was pretty rough in the beginning – I enjoy it more now. We didn't know how successful we would be and we didn't know if we would have enough money. Of course now it is becoming clear that claimants are going to get back close to 100 per cent of their original claim value. So we feel much better about that; it's enjoyable from that aspect' (M. Sheppard, interview, 14 February 1996).

Nevertheless, no system is perfect. Sheppard goes on to say, 'The biggest flaw in the whole thing is that claimants had to have gone to their doctor to get their medical records. For the women that were poor and didn't have medical records ... they were at a disadvantage ... We had to have physical evidence of injury ... That is one of the reasons the Trust came up with the Alternative Dispute Resolution process' (M. Sheppard, interview, 14 February 1996). The ADR referee's decision to offer a decreased award or a zero award usually was based on insufficient evidence provided during the ADR proceedings. Admittedly, the referee's bias sometimes affected the outcome. However, if claimants disagreed with an offer, they could appeal the decision within a sixty-day period.

For Sheppard, the Trust administration and the distribution of funds was successful. In his view, the Trustees were basically motivated to pay the highest amount possible to each individual claimant: 'They understood that fairness was to be maintained throughout the system and that they were not to give the advantage to either the lawyers or groups of lawyers or certain groups of claimants ... There are a lot of people who are happy, and a lot of people who are unhappy, but I think that's what happens when you have to distribute $3 billion' (M. Sheppard, interview, 14 February 1996).

In the final analysis, many will agree with Sybil Shainwald's view that 'This is a very sordid story. What was unsettling about this is that women didn't know about the dangers of the Shield ... I think it was the worst piece of garbage that was ever put on the market and kept on the market purely for profit ... It just ruined hundreds of thousands of women and their family lives ... It added enormously to the health care costs. People looked at what lawyers did and they say lawyers are adding to the cost of the health care budget, but on the other side, I think poor products, bad pharmaceuticals, and bad devices add a tremendous burden to health-care costs, much more than lawyers can ever do' (S. Shainwald, interview, 4 December 1995).

7

Division in the Medical Community

Some physicians did not know how to respond when the news of problems with the Dalkon Shield reached the medical community. Others were perplexed as to how such an apparently dangerous device could have reached the consumer market. Many were sceptical about reports that the Shield was unsafe. Some remained in denial despite U.S. depositories filled with evidence that Dr Hugh Davis and the executives of A.H. Robins knew that the tail string of the Dalkon Shield wicked, causing bacteria to develop in the uterus.

Years of litigation, media coverage, and a multitude of academic studies on the subject still have not convinced some in the medical community that a grave injustice was done to an unsuspecting patient population. Instead, the medical community remains divided over the Dalkon Shield. This division is evident in the numerous journal articles written by physicians between 1970 and 1993, which either concur with or challenge the premise that the Dalkon Shield contributed to hundreds of thousands of women's infertility. However, many of the articles argue that there is a strong association between the Dalkon Shield and pelvic inflammatory disease.

Certain physicians began to draw attention to the Dalkon Shield around the late 1960s and mid-1970s. Dr Howard Tatum reported to the FDA on 25 October 1975 the results of his studies on the Shield. Some of these studies included a comparison of the Shield with several other kinds of IUDs (Tatum 1975b). He specifically examined and compared the tail strings of the various IUDs, and reported his finding that the Dalkon

Shield undoubtedly gathered bacteria within the sheath and spaces of its multifilament tail string (Tatum 1975b). Tatum later wrote several articles that supported his conviction that the Dalkon Shield tail string facilitated bacteria growth that ultimately wicked its way into the uterus (Tatum 1975b, 1975c, 1976).

To explain the validity of his studies during the litigation process, Tatum showed an electronic microscopic image of bacteria growth in the tail string. Photographic images of the same were used in print media and as evidence in the litigation process. Tatum's reputation soon became associated with the Dalkon Shield. In effect, his claim to fame was in providing evidence that the Dalkon Shield tail string had flaws that made it a poor contraceptive.

Although Tatum's theory received support from many other members of the medical community, he also received criticism from some of his peers and eventually from the courts. At the present time, his theory about the wicking of the tail string is no longer used as viable evidence to support a woman's case for injury incurred from the Dalkon Shield. According to Michael Sheppard of the Trust, Tatum's theory is 'junk science' (M. Sheppard, interview, 14 February 1996) (see Appendix A). Similarly, a 1992 article by Drs Stephen Mumford and Elton Kessel claims that the Dalkon Shield had no relationship with PID and was, in fact, a safe contraceptive device (Mumford and Kessel 1992).

According to Dr Carolyn De Marco, 'IUDs increase a woman's risk of PID about twofold, although the risk for modern IUDs is much lower than for older IUDs. This risk is mainly due to the opening of the cervix to insert the IUD' (C. De Marco, interview, 10 October 1995). Dr Bill Freeland suggests that 'labels on IUD packages indicate additional problems in terms of application of the device if put in a nulliparous woman. There are, however, no absolute contraindications. The information is a warning to physicians that the possibility of side effects are more common' (W. Freeland, interview, 23 September 1996).

Others argue that the tail string attached to the Dalkon Shield facilitated the introduction of bacteria into the uterus. Dr Dan Mishell, Jr, presented the view that 'In contrast to the loop and the copper IUDs, which have a monofilament tail string, the Shield has a multifilament tail string. Studies in both human beings and animals have shown that this type of appendage provides a means for bacteria to ascend to the upper genital tract during the entire time the IUD is in place and thus increases the risk of salpingitis [inflammation of the fallopian tubes]' (Mishell 1985, 985).

In the past, women were sometimes judged on a moral level by their physicians. Many doctors supported the notion that sexually transmitted diseases such as chlamydia and gonorrhea led women who had more than one sexual partner to incur infertility. Today, some physicians describe the term 'promiscuity' in biological terms rather than moral ones. As Dr Paul Claman explains, 'The problem is that promiscuity sounds like a value judgment ... People have more than one relationship in modern society. So, when we speak about promiscuity we are talking more of the biological issue of transmission of sexually transmitted diseases, which can happen' (P. Claman, interview, 22 November 1995).

On the other hand, one does not need to have had more than one sexual partner to be at risk for a sexually transmitted disease. It is, in fact, one's sexual behaviour that may alter the natural defence mechanisms of a healthy body. Evidence shows that specific sexual behaviour within a monogamous relationship may facilitate contracting PID or chlamydia. For instance, anal intercourse followed by vaginal intercourse can transfer bacteria from one area to the other. Likewise, bacteria can be introduced if a woman uses talcum powder or tampons (A. Leader, interview, 27 November 1995). Dr Norman Barwin states, 'One way one gets PID is through sperm. Sperm are the carriers ... so the contaminated sperm tracks up the IUD string and ... the set up is there' (N. Barwin, interview, 20 October 1995). In other words, if a man has contracted PID, it is likely that he will pass it on to a sexual partner through his sperm.

Most doctors agree that many IUDs should not be inserted in a woman who has not been pregnant, has had an episode of PID or sexually transmitted disease, or has or had more than one sexual partner. Some claim that the best candidate for an IUD is a woman who has had children and is in a monogamous relationship – this assumes that her partner is also monogamous. In these instances, the risk of pelvic infection or sexually transmitted disease is decreased. Unfortunately, many women who used the Dalkon Shield had never been pregnant or had a history of one infection or another.

Many of the articles written on the Dalkon Shield or other IUDs address the possibility of one or two of the above-described variables being a possible culprit in causing infertility or PID. Mumford and Kessel (1992, 1151) asserted that a 'physician's skill and experience is far more important to successful IUD insertion than previously recognized.'

Other medical studies have presented the potential problems of IUDs, including those associated with the Dalkon Shield. For example, a study conducted in 1991 concluded that the 'use of the Dalkon Shield has been found to be associated with an increased risk of primary tubal infertility ... The risk of PID associated with the Dalkon Shield may have been related to the design of its multifilament string' (Washington et al. 1991, 266). The authors also found that 'despite 25 studies conducted worldwide, the link between the rise of intrauterine devices (IUDs) and the development of PID remains one of the most controversial topics in contemporary contraception' (Washington et al. 1991, 18). Buchan et al. concluded that 'among women currently using an IUD (of any kind), those who had used a Dalkon Shield (at any time) had nearly five times as great a risk of hospital referral for pelvic inflammatory disease as those who had never used a Dalkon Shield' (1990, 780). Daling et al. also concluded in 1985 that 'use of the Dalkon Shield (and possibly of plastic IUDs other than those that contain copper) can lead to infertility in nulligravid [never had a pregnancy] women' (1985, 312). Grimes's (1987) article concluded that 'the Dalkon Shield appears associated with a higher risk of pelvic inflammatory disease than the Lippes Loop, Saf-T-Coil, or copper devices' (p. 97). Vessey et al. (1981) stated that acute definite disease occurred somewhat more frequently during the early months of the use of an IUD than during the later months; the highest rate (8.1 per 1000 woman-years) was observed in users of the Dalkon Shield (p. 855). Finally, Marshall et al.'s 1974 study reported that in 296 nonindigent nulliparous women using the Dalkon Shield, the pregnancy and medical removal rates calculated at the end of twelve months were 5.6 and 28.7, respectively, per 100 women. Dr David Eschenbach supported these views on IUDs in general: 'The IUD is a potential threat to future fertility. Tubal infertility is caused by a prior episode of pelvic inflammatory disease (PID). For women who have never been pregnant, prior IUD use increases tubal infertility two- to sixfold (200% to 600%) (1–3)' (Eschenbach 1992, 1177). Clearly, a number of physicians concurred that the Dalkon Shield did not represent a safe contraceptive device.

Conversely, Snowden and Pearson (1984), Davis (1970), Ostergard (1973), Mumford and Kessel (1992), and Rioux (1993) maintain that pelvic inflammatory disease was not a result of the structure of the Dalkon Shield's tail string. They argue that the Shield was a safe contraceptive device and that other factors played an integral role in causing PID in Dalkon Shield users.

Snowden and Pearson's (1984) analysis of reports of PID possibly related to four common IUDs in 1971 to 1978 in Britain led them to conclude that 'fears that the Dalkon Shield may be associated with a higher incidence of pelvic infection than other intrauterine devices may have been unjustified.' In the same article, the authors stated that 'the timing of fitting, and the wearer, suggests that any observed differences in reported infection rates are due to variables other than the type of intrauterine device fitted' (p. 1570).

Dr Donald R. Ostergard reported that 'the device is well tolerated and has a low expulsion rate and medical removal rates. The pregnancy rate of 1.2 per cent remained constant after 12 months of use' (1973, p. 1088 abstract). Ostergard also continued to insist that the nulliparous model Dalkon Shield proved to be an effective IUD for women who had never had a pregnancy.

Around the same time, Dr Hugh Davis, the inventor of the Dalkon Shield, concluded that 'expulsion and removals for bleeding complications have been greatly reduced with the modern Shield type of IUD, yielding continuation rates distinctly superior to barrier methods, oral contraceptives or the older types of intrauterine device in general use' (Davis 1970, 455). Later, Davis indicated in a 1972 article that complications associated with large-scale use of IUDs were associated more with technical lapses during insertion, or were merely coincidental gynecological complaints. He warned that the 'method cannot be considered a universal panacea. Every physician is not skilled in the use of the devices, nor is every woman a suitable candidate for the method' (Davis 1972, 149–50). In the early 1970s Davis had presented guidelines for the use and consequences of the Dalkon Shield.

Some years later, other physicians supported and reiterated similar guidelines to the medical community via journal articles. Canadian Dr Jacques Rioux wrote, 'We have few but good IUDs. Their use after proper patient selection (choosing the right woman), careful counseling (good programme support), gentle insertion at the fundus (delicate and proper technique) will result in effective and safe contraception' (Rioux 1993, 924). He championed the Dalkon Shield as well as other IUDs. In doing so, Rioux emphasized, like Mumford and Kessel, that because the Dalkon Shield was a difficult device to insert only very experienced physicians should do so and only in a specific patient population. In contrast, Dr Brian Ivey, a British physician residing in Canada, commented that the manufacturer produced a marketing film to show how the Shield should be inserted. Ivey emphasized, 'You saw the device being advanced before the cervix and then a frame later the device had gone and the applicator was being removed. It didn't show the effect ... It was supposed to be a Cadillac, well, I think like a lot of Cadillacs, it was over-priced and over-advertised' (B. Ivey, interview, 22 September 1995).

Drs Stephen Mumford and Elton Kessel questioned whether the science underlying the indictment of the Dalkon Shield was sound. They also questioned the research methodologies of those who challenged the safety of the Dalkon Shield. Mumford and Kessel presented these and other questions in a 1992 paper in which they examined numerous Dalkon Shield reviews. In particular, they vehemently criticized the numerous case-controlled studies that resulted in negative perceptions of the Dalkon Shield. The authors felt that these biases may have accounted for specific conflicts among the results of randomized studies. Many of the reports examined suggested that the Dalkon Shield resulted in a higher rate of PID than other IUDs. They concluded that the indictment of the Dalkon Shield was a mistake, and that other variables influenced the development of PID in Dalkon Shield users.

Dr David Eschenbach's views differed somewhat from those of Mumford and Kessel. He wrote, 'First, and most important, is the recognition that the IUD causes pelvic inflammatory disease (PID). Lay people, first year medical students, and most physicians recognize that foreign bodies placed in the human body have a propensity to cause infection' (Eschenbach 1992, 1178). Eschenbach concluded that reviews of the Dalkon Shield by Mumford, Kessel, and Kronmal 'presented such a one-sided view that they are best termed extensive editorials' (p. 1178). He also noted that in Mumford and Kessel's review, 'Case-studies are summarily dismissed, although they represent the only controlled data where the risk of PID is compared with users of other or no contraceptives ... The longitudinal clinical trials of IUDs were designed to examine several issues but none was adequately designed to diagnose diligently or record PID' (p. 1179). Eschenbach makes the valid argument that one methodology cannot be dismissed for another when attempting to arrive at viable answers to health-related questions.

Admittedly, the aforementioned studies are only a small sample of the diverse views among medical practitioners about the Dalkon Shield, IUDs, and PID. However, several of these authors had reviewed studies that incorporated a cross-section of investigative studies by prominent physicians and researchers in the medical field. Their conclusions, therefore, are based on substantive data produced by respected professionals. It is crucial to learn from all the different perspectives presented and to remember that randomized studies united with case-control studies provide a richer body of evidence. Many agree that several variables contributed to the infections that women suffered while using the Dalkon Shield.

A portion of North American gynecologists claim that they were not aware of problems with the Shield because they were too busy with their practices to read the numerous medical articles, newsletters, and government notifications that warned of its dangers. Dr Dorothy Shaw argues, 'I wonder about the expectation that we have of the average family physician. When you think about what has happened to medicine, we know that a significant amount of what is learned ten years prior is obsolete. It is a constant educational venture. Physicians try hard to keep up with increasing changes' (D. Shaw, interview, 16 October 1995). Many Dalkon Shield survivors do not accept this as a valid excuse. Lack of knowledge or undecided views about the Shield are no doubt part of the reason why some physicians took a defensive position when it came to assisting female patients who alleged that they were infected by the Shield. Dr Brian Ivey remarked, 'I stopped using the Dalkon Shield before it was withdrawn, purely because I didn't like it as a device to be used. It was difficult to put in ... It also looked like something that should be at the other end of a fishing line' (B. Ivey, interview, 22 September 1995).

Physicians wrote to A.H. Robins and the FDA asking for advice on what they should do. Others complained that there was no way they could contact, in some cases, a total of 6,000 or more patients. As a rule, Planned Parenthood or community clinics often had patients that visited only once, never to be seen again. As a result, physicians did not always know how to contact these patients of the early 1970s. Some physicians expressed the sentiment, 'In most cases, it had been ten or fifteen years prior that some patients had the Shield inserted. What were we supposed to do?'

Correspondence from lawyers put most physicians in a panic. Dr Norman Barwin states, 'I think a lot of physicians felt the threat of litigation, and feared being implicated ... A person who actually inserted this thinks, well, if I get involved in this I may be accused of it' (N. Barwin, interview, 20 October 1995). On the other hand, when physicians received requests from lawyers for claimants' medical records, the requests usually informed them that they would not be implicated in the Dalkon Shield litigation. In other words, the physicians' fear of malpractice suits was unfounded.

The panic that went through the medical community is evident in the A.H. Robins correspondence available through the U.S. Freedom of Access to Information Act. Responses to physicians' inquiries about the removal of the Shield were similar to the following letter excerpt, dated 19 December 1980 from the Director of Medical Services of A.H. Robins:

Dear Dr

Thank you very much for your letter of December 4, 1989, regarding our September 25 'Dear doctor' letter regarding removal of the Dalkon Shield. I am not aware of any specific methods or means available to us which would assist physicians to identify and locate patients who might still have the device ... If among your patients there are a substantial number who do not routinely come in for periodic checkups and who you feel will not be reached by various media reports, you may wish to consider a chart review for the identification and notification of such patients to come in for a checkup. It should be fairly easy to separate out those who seek regular follow-up care ... We will be willing to consider some support for the necessary secretarial services. We would appreciate your estimate of the costs incident to such a review before making a final commitment ...

Sincerely,
Fletcher B. Owen, Jr, MD, PhD
Director of Medical Services (A.H. Robins)

These types of replies did not always alleviate the physicians' concerns. In 1980, physicians were confused and unsure about the extent of their liability. Even if A.H. Robins and, much later, the Dalkon Shield Claimants Trust attempted to assure them that they were absolved of any responsibility, physicians still had sleepless nights.

Most physicians felt obligated to contact as many patients as possible for removal of the Shield. The doctors interviewed for this book underlined that most physicians felt badly about the tragedy that struck many of the women who had used the Dalkon Shield. Some lost faith in the medical studies presented in medical journals. The Dalkon Shield saga has also lowered the reputation of some research institutions. The repercussions of the Shield have left many scars on both the consumer and the medical community. A measure of this concern is reflected in more frequent examination of drug and medical device regulations and policy in the United States and Canada.

Some physicians agree that money, politics, and big pharmaceutical companies play a role in which contraceptives are marketed. 'According to a study conducted by the Canadian Public Health Association, drug companies spend ... $10,000 annually per physician, on marketing and promotion' (Parsons and Parsons 1995, 92). Physicians are routinely asked by pharmaceutical representatives to participate in clinical studies to test medical products. In the 1970s and 1980s it was not unusual for pharmaceutical companies to offer perks to physicians, such as a computer or a vacation, if they agreed to take part in a clinical trial (Parsons and Parsons 1995). The patient received free drugs or a free device for the duration of the study. However, afterwards the patient was expected to pay. 'The most serious breach of ethics by doctors engaged in these studies is the difficulty that they sometimes have in gaining patient participation without making the patient feel coerced' (Parsons and Parsons 1995, 94). This supports reports from some Dalkon Shield survivors that they felt coerced or intimidated into continuing to use the Shield despite their complaints of pain. However, 'Doctors are becoming increasingly wary of drug companies and their approaches to research and marketing and the relationship between the two' (Parsons and Parsons 1995, 96). Regulations established by Health Canada's Medical Devices Bureau are presently under examination. These regulations are addressed in Chapter 9.

Dr Marion Powell maintains, 'We'd had a lot of problems with IUDs in the 1960s and so when the Dalkon Shield came along it appeared to answer some of the problems we had, such as expulsion. So, in light of the frustration we had, the Dalkon Shield seemed to be a good answer ... So, you have to look at the Dalkon Shield in the context of what had gone on ahead of it and what was happening later. Later, we were much more selective about who got IUDs' (M. Powell, interview, 8 August 1995).

Dr David Eschenbach (1992) firmly stated in an editorial that women must be informed of the potential risk of PID and sterility from using IUDs. He further said that the IUD facilitates the development of PID in patients who have sexually transmitted diseases. Nevertheless, PID can also occur in the first four to six months after insertion of an IUD. Therefore, the use of antibiotics in selected patients should be studied. Eschenbach suggested that long-time users of IUDs are at risk for abscesses because bacteria grows in a biofilm layer on the string and the body of the IUD. Ultimately, Eschenbach advised that physicians 'need to stop trying to fool themselves in the case of IUD infection – it is not some abstract concept. The universal recognition and teaching of this fact will prompt increased physician and patient surveillance for infection before tubal occlusion' (p. 1178).

Ultimately, we need to consider the growing perspective that a holistic investigative approach is needed when attempting to determine what is best for the patient. Furthermore, examining government regulations past and present may offer some insights as to whether changes have occurred in institutional arenas that determine the validity of medical devices and drugs. Follow-up research is crucial to identifying the lessons learned from the Dalkon Shield. According to Eschenbach, 'There has been no new data published on the risk of PID among women with the Dalkon Shield since 1985' (Eschenbach 1992, 1178). This lapse of time is inordinately long for such an important area of study.

As emphasized by several physicians in different ways, 'We go into medicine to heal, not to harm' (P. Claman, interview, 22 November 1995). However, 'The fact is that drug companies are in business to make money ... So what we are left with is the fact we have to place a good deal of responsibility for maintaining the ethical purity of these encounters on the shoulders of the doctors' (Parsons and Parsons 1995, 95). The question remains about whether it is fair for doctors to shoulder all of the responsibility.

8
Lessons Learned and Not Learned

The Dalkon Shield, Thalidomide, and DES became metaphors in our culture, but they have never said, 'How could this have occurred?' Many of these issues like this we are not very good at revisiting.
Madelaine Bosco, 16 January 1995

Human nature seems to resist reading and learning from history – hence, the same mistakes tend to get repeated all too often.
Dr Nedra R. Lander, 14 May 1996

Probably the main lesson learned from the Dalkon Shield tragedy is that IUDs are not a good form of contraceptive for women who have not had a child – the risk of infection and possible infertility is too high. Nor should IUDs be used by women who have more than one sexual partner. Moreover, if a man has more than one sexual partner he should not engage in sexual relations with a woman who uses an IUD; in doing so, he puts the woman's health at risk. Further, IUDs can be agents for PID or sexually transmitted disease no matter how the infection was contracted: women using any IUD can be infected through a variety of means, whether it is through a medical procedure, sexual activity, or a design flaw in the IUD.

Conversely, the best candidate for any IUD is a woman who is in a relationship in which she and her sexual partner are faithful to each other. Moreover, this woman must have a physician who is skilled in inserting IUDs and is up to date about the pros and cons of various contraceptive methods. The chosen physician must also be concerned about and aware of the patient's needs and lifestyle so as to advise her appropriately about her health-care needs. Consumers must also educate themselves about appropriate health-care treatments and choices.

Dalkon Shield survivors have learned that women must trust their own instincts about their health. They must listen to what their bodies are telling them. If a woman is experiencing pain from an IUD or any internal medical device, then she should not hesitate to have it removed. If a physician refuses to remove it, she should find one who will.

During the 1970s and 1980s, many users of the Dalkon Shield assumed their physicians knew best. Some of these women suffered through excruciating pain for an intolerable length of time for no good reason. Eventually, many of them learned to take charge of their health, which meant finding a doctor who would remove the Shield and listen and react sensitively to them. It meant the women trusting their own instincts, becoming aware of how their bodies functioned, and attending to their own pain. Nancy, a Dalkon Shield survivor, reflects, 'I used to think that doctors were gods. I would listen to them, but I will never do that again. I also will never put a foreign object into my body again' (Nancy, interview, 24 October 1995). Likewise, Eileen stated, 'I've learned mankind in general is off-base. The real main lesson is that there isn't anything you can count on. It's not going to change out there' (Eileen, interview, 24 October 1995).

Basically, one must consider several issues surrounding one's health. Survivors advise interviewing a doctor before deciding if that doctor will consider your interests and serve your health needs, values, and belief system. Compatible values between the doctor and the patient are crucial to the integrity of the relationship (N.R. Lander, interview, 14 May 1996).

During the 1970s, both physicians and patients were ignorant of the Dalkon Shield's potential harm. Many physicians accepted information from pharmaceutical companies and literature about the Dalkon Shield at face value. Their patients thus placed a great deal of trust in the doctor's decision-making powers. In essence, the relationship between the physician and the patient during this time was hierarchical – the physician told the patient what to do and the patient usually complied. Today, doctors are more aware of the potential for a malpractice suit because of the increase in personal injury lawsuits, particularly in the United

States. As well, patients are more assertive about standing up for their rights.

Since doctors don't have all the answers, treatment should be a shared decision between doctor and patient. This approach would involve listening to anecdotal accounts of symptoms and devising an agreeable and realistic method of treatment for the patient. Taking an extra ten minutes with a patient may avoid undue risks to her or his health, as well as reduce the pressure on the doctor to take on all the responsibility. Perhaps the lesson learned here is that the hierarchical model no longer works for patients or doctors.

Dr Paul Claman agrees: 'I think in the past we didn't have a lot to offer in terms of effective intervention. We played more the part of the Shaman. In a sense we had more power, as healers. The relationship the Shaman has with the patient, by definition, is to be paternalistic. I think medicine has changed a lot ... The young doctors are now being versed in interaction with their patients and have them participate in making decisions about their care. I think that is new. Part of this is because of the Dalkon Shield' (P. Claman, interview, 22 November 1995).

According to Dr Marion Powell, the events surrounding the Dalkon Shield have made physicians much more critical of literature reviews. However, 'There is still far too much accepting of everything that comes out' (M. Powell, interview, 28 August 1995). Nevertheless, some physicians are less likely to accept products from pharmaceutical sales representatives. Moreover, teaching physicians now recognize the importance of encouraging medical students to ask questions. Dr Brian Ivey points out,

I think the corporate body of experience of the medical profession and now both at the official level and practical level are a little dubious about new medications ... I also think that a lot of things that have perhaps come out of this is that patients will realize the individual physicians were not necessarily any better informed than they were ... We rely on what we are told and our experience. I also think certain good things come out of bad things. There is a greater awareness to avoid claims of excellence ... Unfortunately, the people [who have gained this] experience ... have lost a lot more on an individual basis for which they can never be adequately compensated. (B. Ivey, interview, 22 September 1995)

Opinions offered by some physicians seem to indicate a recognition that changes in the way medicine is practised are needed. According to one study on doctor/patient relations, 'Today, patients are arriving at their doctors' offices armed with "amazing" amounts of knowledge and high expectations ... some will come in and they've gone through the internet. They have very pointed questions, very smart questions' (Kirkey 1996).

Dr Pierre Blais, a biologist, advises consumers not to believe everything they are told, especially by a doctor: 'Consider your physician as a contractor. He or she is at the same plane as a mechanic who is assigned to fixing your car.' Blais's insights are garnered from his experience with government, pharmaceutical companies, and physicians. He worked with Health and Welfare Canada in the 1970s and 1980s during the initial warnings about the Dalkon Shield and breast implants, and today works in the United States in research and analysis of implants. 'The education of the physician in connection with the drugs and the devices he or she prescribes may be no more than what you have. The physician was educated from the salesperson ... You would not buy a car without getting the operators' manual' (P. Blais, interview, 12 August 1995).

Blais urges consumers to insist on what by mandate, and in some cases by law, the physician must provide – research information on products. 'The Dalkon Shield has been revisited on three occasions: the Copper 7, breast implants, and female and male lars joints have all had adverse reactions – the damage has been greater than the Shield ... If the consumers do not learn how to seek education voluntarily and habitually, we will have a fourth one. We do not have the resources to protect us from this type of fiasco. You are on your own. You are responsible for your health.' Blais also warns that government and industry have not learned any lessons from the Dalkon Shield or breast implants. He predicts that the next medical device disaster will focus on surgical procedures and faulty surgical instruments. However, he does not believe that anyone will heed his warnings since, in the 1970s, no one in the U.S. Food and Drug Administration or the Canadian Health Protection Branch regarded his warnings about the Dalkon Shield. Blais later set off alarms about the dangers of breast implants. He was then fired from the federal government because of, according to him, his opposition to such products and because his objections were seen as disruptive. Blais was later reinstated, yet chose to resign voluntarily (P. Blais, interview, 12 August 1995). He is not alone in his views – physicians, patients, and lawyers interviewed for this book warn that governments and medical and legal systems do not have provisions in place to safeguard our welfare. The message that consumers must increase their knowledge for their own safety is constant in the stories of past and recent health-care tragedies.

Women who used the Dalkon Shield and who were advised to have a hysterectomy later wondered if it was necessary. Dr Carolyn DeMarco maintains that, even today, surgical procedures such as hysterectomies and mastectomies are still unnecessarily prescribed: 'We have horrible procedures being committed on women every day. Most recently, there are unnecessary Caesarean sections. For example, a repeat Caesarean section is a two to four times greater risk for the mother than a vaginal birth ... We also have coronary bypass surgery, which is very costly. If anything, I would have hoped that the Dalkon Shield [aftermath] would have questioned not only devices, but surgery procedures and untested drugs' (C. DeMarco, interview, 10 October 1995).

Many of the survivors who joined forces with activist groups learned that working together to achieve justice had its benefits. Together, they could direct public attention to the issue. The experience taught them that there can be solace for those who are able to reach out. It gave the women a sense of camaraderie and community in helping others, and relieved many of the sense of isolation. Activist Deanne stated, 'One thing I learned was that you are never alone with anything. There is always someone out there feeling what you are feeling. One of the healing processes is being lucky enough to find those people and compare and share notes. I looked around and thanked God I had met these women because they suddenly made me realize that I'm a strong person' (Deanne, interview, 24 October 1995).

Unfortunately, one of the lessons some women learned is that there will always be someone seeking to gain from other people's misery. Laura Jones wrote this letter:

After analyzing my feelings, I realize that from the second A.H. Robins was sold and the Trust was in place, I don't believe lawyers should have been involved at all. Lawyers further victimized DS survivors. What we needed in this process was a sense of empowerment, of taking charge, of feeling some control over what was going on. There was nothing to prove. We had to gather all our medical records and fill out a form. There was lots of room for an anecdotal history which was much better written by the DS wearer than the lawyer. The best lawyers in the world couldn't argue medical records that showed that other IUDs were worn. Any woman that said, 'I needed help getting medical records etc.' could have got that information from the Trust and other DS women. By that time, it was relatively easy to get in contact with other DS women. But my experience was that somehow we didn't really believe that other DS women could know more than the lawyers – the social conditioning is so strong. (L. Jones, 22 April 1996)

A lesson many lawyers learned is that the court system has the last word. They also learned that the bottom line in winning such cases is often based on dollars and cents. As lawyer Robert Montague put it, '[O]ur courts generally have a funny idea on the value of human life' (R. Montague, interview, 17 August 1995). On the other hand, lawyer Mike Pretl claims, 'One cannot expect a system like this to run sensitively and satisfy people's personal needs ... If you are handling that amount of money in what is apparently an adversarial process you are going to end up being adversarial and not sensitive' (M. Pretl, interview, 27 October 1996).

The entire litigation process has awakened some lawyers to the multifaceted nature of the law and of human nature and has introduced a newfound cynicism into their thinking. One lawyer aptly stated that the last ten years made him realize that law is not a place where you can have justice. Other lawyers confided that they do not believe it is possible to find objective truth because most people find facts to support their own positions. Most frustrating was the experience of trying to prove the survivors' cases. Some lawyers advised that to decrease this element of frustration in such cases for the client and the lawyer that women and men must get copies of their medical records on an annual basis. One lawyer stated that he now has his wife retrieve copies of her medical records regularly. His reasoning: 'Someday we may want to prove something' (Anonymous, interview, 1995).

For many lawyers, the experience of interacting with women who had incurred injuries from the Dalkon Shield increased their empathy with women's experiences. Carey Linde stated, 'All I can say is that it was an educational experience in which I would like to think that the empathy I picked up made me a better person as a male in society' (C. Linde, interview, 12 September 1995). Finally, most lawyers commented that they and most of their clients have learned that one must critically challenge any information that professes to be the last word.

Madelaine Bosco, a health educator and policy-maker with the Winnipeg Health Clinic, opposes using civil litigation to punish those who produce and market harmful products: 'I have a problem with civil litigation as a punishment of people. It is based on "You are the bad guy, so you have to pay $10,000" instead of "You are the bad guy, and you should serve time" ... Why aren't they in jail?' She further points out that generally people do not listen despite large lawsuits and the billions of dollars paid out to claimants: 'In fact, it happened and it was business as usual. I look at industry to have learned from it. For example, let's look at our own shop and make sure it doesn't happen again. This, of course, hasn't occurred ... Pharmaceutical manufacturers are pressuring the FDA to allow more room for drugs and devices to be marketed to the public ... The Canadian Medical Devices Bureau is no further ahead in yielding to the same pressures' (M. Bosco, interview, 20 April 1996).

Lawyer John Baker adds, 'Unfortunately, I think the sins of the A.H. Robins company would be easier to commit now. The pharmaceutical companies in the U.S. will find it easier to commit those types of frauds because there is a movement in the government to deregulate the industry. This movement for deregulation has caused a significant weakening of the FDA's ability to prevent another Dalkon Shield catastrophe' (J. Baker, interview, 14 November 1996). Likewise, lawyer and former judge Miles Lord states, 'The FDA is going to turn that stuff loose and not test it ... We have learned nothing about controlling pharmaceutical products. In fact, the scare that was thrown into the pharmaceutical companies has caused them to build up fortifications against any criticism whatsoever ... They do it by buying politicians' (M. Lord, interview, 15 April 1996). Such statements suggest that tragedies such as the Dalkon Shield have made no impression upon government officials or industry.

Many of the lessons not learned continue to haunt us in the aftermath of the Dalkon Shield. 'We know much about the tragic experience of these women here and abroad, yet here in the U.S. there are still young poor women today who are encouraged to use contraceptives that produce devastating results to their bodies and their lives' (M. Lord, interview, 16 April 1996). As well, contraceptives are still exported to some under-developed countries to be tested on poor women (Akhter 1995).

A 1996 CBC television documentary entitled 'The Human Labora-tory' described the plight of such women who were using the Norplant contraceptive device. This is a rod-like device, which looks like a small matchstick, that is placed underneath the skin of the arm. Farida Akhter reports that women in Bangladesh who used Norplant complained of loss of vision, dizziness, and continuous bleeding from the vagina (Akhter 1995). Women were experiencing such adverse side-effects that they visited clinics twelve to fifteen times before finding a doctor who would remove the device. In most cases, it was not removed at all. In many cases if it was removed, the woman was treated horribly. Medical anthropologist Catherine Maternowska, who worked with physicians in Haiti, recounts one example: 'One woman came to have [the Norplant implant] removed and the doctor said, "Look, she is an animal." He threw her on the table and before the anaesthetic could take effect they started taking it out. The skin and muscle sinew had grown over it. The woman was wailing' (CBC 1996). In this same documentary, North American women with the Norplant device were shown suffering dizzi-ness, frequent bleeding, and impaired vision. Yet one woman stated that after one year of pain, the problems disappeared. She decided to keep the device for its convenience and hope for the best.

Women's groups suggest that population control organizations aim to decrease world population by imposing unsafe contraceptives on poor and uneducated women. These organizations suggest that women's groups are unconcerned about how quickly the world population is growing. Margaret Catley-Carlson, President of the Population Council (a U.S. organization concerned with policy and issues related to popula-tion control), stated in July 1993, 'The Norplant implant is not a perfect method, but it is a good one. It is not every woman's choice, but it is the choice of many' (Akhter 1995, 11). Farida Akhter argues, 'The Popula-tion Council ... know very well that these women are deprived of their right to choose the means of survival ... They are given false promises and information. They are cheated' (Akhter 1995, 11). Similarly, a contraceptive called Quinacrine has recently been promoted in underdeveloped countries. This injectable 'contraceptive' pellet works by creating scar tissue in the fallopian tubes, thereby encouraging permanent infertility. Although not yet approved by the FDA, Drs Stephen Mumford and Elton Kessel, who argued that the Dalkon Shield was safe, maintain in the same CBC documentary that Quinacrine will assist in population control. Mumford states in the program, 'Women want this; there are a lot of grateful women' (CBC 1996).

Dr Amy Pollack, Medical Director of the International Association for Voluntary Surgical Contraception (AVSC), states in the documentary 'The Human Laboratory' that Quinacrine has not been approved for over 100,000 women worldwide, yet these women have been told it is a safe contraceptive. 'Two men are running around the world with a suitcase full of pills ... the prime appeal is low cost' (CBC 1996).

When the Chair of Global Population Concerns of Ottawa, Madeline Weld, was asked to comment about the content of 'The Human Laboratory,' she said that she did not have the full facts on Quinacrine, nor was she up to date on the numbers of women affected by Norplant, so she could not comment. However, she did venture to say, 'I do not agree with those women who are trying to stop research on [these products]' (CBC 1996). Weld also remarked, 'If there is something cheap, why should we be against it if it is ethical, safe and properly tested?' (M. Weld, interview, 7 May 1996). At the same time Weld wrote in an article, 'Is investment in female education really the best way to slow population growth? ... Should we put all the available money into the education of girls at the expense of meeting the family-planning needs of their mothers and big sisters? The answer is NO' (Weld 1996). However, Weld later stated that 'The women in question should be informed that [Norplant or any inserted device] will prevent pregnancy and it works in such and such a way. If they are in pain, they should be able to have it removed ... I think drug companies should be regulated. They shouldn't be allowed to dump things on the third world that are considered unsafe in our country' (M. Weld, interview, 7 May 1996).

Hundreds of lawsuits have been launched against American Home Products, the manufacturer of Norplant, claiming such injuries as memory loss, autoimmune disorder, seizures, and blindness. In 1994, a class action lawsuit on behalf of women who claimed that Dow Corning's silicone breast implants had injured them was settled with a payment of $4.25 billion – the largest ever. However, by September 1995 the settlement was in danger of collapsing. In addition, a class action lawsuit has been filed on behalf of men with penile implants. It has been suggested by activist groups and some lawyers that certain lawyers are trawling for silicone implant business and advertising for clients who have ever used a medical device ('On the needless ...' 1995). Similar allegations were directed at lawyers involved in the Dalkon Shield cases. Are these allegations just another form of deflecting attention away from the real issue of questionable medical devices?

People who had silicone breast implants are still being denied full recognition of their injuries. Dow Corning, which marketed the implants, denies deceiving the public. Chair and CEO of Dow Corning, Richard Hazeldon, argues that the FDA Commissioner, Dr David Kessler, stated before the U.S. Congress that Mayo Clinic and Harvard University studies on breast implants were based on good science that provides reassurance that there is not a large risk of women developing autoimmune disease from the implants relative to women who do not have such implants (NBC 1995).

However, John Swanson, a former executive of Dow Corning and husband of a breast implant survivor, pointed out that the FDA Commissioner also stated that the manufacturer had not yet proved the product to be safe (NBC 1995). Swanson also stated that corporate memos documenting certain aspects about the breast implants coincidentally disappeared when some CEOs of Dow had been notified that an investigation might be pending. Similarly, documents at A.H. Robins about the Dalkon Shield had disappeared prior to an investigation. A former A.H. Robins attorney, Roger Tuttle, testified that general counsel William Forrest had ordered Tuttle to arrange the destruction of Shield documents (Mintz 1985). Investigations into A.H. Robins' activities and more recently into Dow Corning's led both companies to file for Chapter 11 bankruptcy as protection from financial ruin. Dow's move to reorganize its assets was again similar to the A.H. Robins reorganization plan. To date, 191,000 claims have been filed against Dow Corning.

In both the Dalkon Shield and breast implant scenarios, women were told that the devices had a high degree of safety, despite the findings of independent research studies. Women who filed claims against the companies were humiliated with inappropriate questions about their personal behaviour and credibility. In both scenarios, government regulations have not protected women or men from the risks related to these products. Apparently, physicians still buy into pharmaceutical companies' marketing, and consumers still allow themselves to be manipulated by seductive imagery and rhetoric.

9

Aftermath, Recommendations, and Conclusions

Why does this book revisit the Dalkon Shield story? The value of re-examining such tragedies lies in the insights they give us into the dynamics of medical research, practices, and values; corporations' profit motives; and the justice system.

The multiple effects of the Dalkon Shield range from the economic to the social, emotional, physical, and spiritual. If we consider the tragic repercussions of the Shield, we may be able to devise ways to decrease the risk of other harmful products reaching the market. The following recommendations are based on interviews with and correspondence from claimants, physicians, lawyers, and others.

Physicians need to consider their historic role as healers in a society now dominated by new technologies. Paramount to this consideration is examining their relationship with pharmaceutical companies. For example, how much do doctors know about these companies' research practices, promotional strategies, profit margins, and health-care agendas? Do doctors' prescription practices knowingly or unwittingly support the pharmaceutical companies' means of sustaining their economic growth? Do doctors support research studies in exchange for gifts? In light of these questions, physicians must consider their own value systems. Also, they need to examine whether their knowledge of a pharmaceutical product is based mainly on the reports, sales skills, and perks offered by sales representatives rather than on articles published in independent, peer-reviewed medical journals.

It is vital to the overall socio-economic costs of the health-care system that doctors establish and sustain trusting and ethical relationships with their patients. Part of this involves suspending moral judgments about a patient, as well as abiding by an important part of the Hippocratic oath, 'Do no harm.'

It is also recommended that doctors not yield to the pressures of the present administrative, political, and economic factors involved in health-care reform. To this end, an anonymous distress telephone line for health-care workers having difficulty coping with the mounting stresses in the present health-care environment should be established. A similar, community-funded, distress line has been available for general public use for a number of years. Another possibility is access to a confidential Internet distress line for health-care professionals.

Physicians and hospital staff could also implement a risk assessment and risk management model on all fronts of health care as a proactive stance against unwarranted injury or disease. Scholarly Canadian physicians must abide by the statement of principles of the Society for Social Responsibility in Science ('Ethics for scientific researchers' 1971). In brief, this statement recommends that scholarly physicians should foresee the results of their professional work, assume moral responsibility for their work, put effort into work that will benefit humanity, and share their scientific knowledge and ethical judgments with government and laypeople. Likewise, according to a recent statement made by the President of the American Medical Association, Dr L.R. Bristow, on a television broadcast, practising physicians should 'continue to honour the social contract that we made with the public twenty-four centuries ago with our code of ethics. That code of ethics says that we will never do anything that takes advantage of the vulnerable patient' (Global TV Network 1996).

Finally, doctors must consider past tragedies, like that of the Dalkon Shield, when recommending any drug or device to a patient. As one doctor said, 'I took one look at [the Dalkon Shield] and decided I would not use it' (P. Tremblay, interview, 1995). Thus, physicians must trust their own instincts when making a decision about patient care.

Needless to say, educating our future health professionals about the Dalkon Shield and other disastrous medical products is vital. Medical students in particular need to be made aware of their moral and legal accountability. At present, medical students examine case studies or reviews of historical cases. They also receive lectures on the topic of contraception. The history of IUDs and other contraceptives should be part of seminar classes on contraception and medical ethics for students to analyse critically and discuss. To this end, people who have been involved in such cases as that of the Dalkon Shield could be invited to give guest lectures. Invitations could also be extended to public health nurses or health advocacy leaders to lecture on the importance of critically analysing reviews of new medical products. In brief, medical schools need to involve others in the health-care arena to provide their alternative and experiential insights.

Evaluation of medical students' interpersonal skills should be mandatory throughout their years in medical school. Their interaction style and responsiveness to patients need to be closely monitored. Sensitivity training on diverse cultural values, beliefs, and attitudes should be part of this process. Bias awareness seminars could be available within a medical curriculum or as part of an internship program. These courses would help to inform students of their own prejudices, values, biases, or lack of information about other people.

Health education, however, needs to start in high school, particularly education on safe and effective contraceptive methods, safe sex, and similar topics that allow students to make responsible and informed choices.

According to Dr William Freeland, Chief of the Devices Evaluation Division of the Health Protection Branch, Health Canada, 'In 1995 many of the hazardous medical devices are not left in the body. We are trying to get regulations which will allow us to continue updates on risks of a device ... If we had been smart in the 1970s or the government had been sufficiently involved in the 1970s, the ability to identify risks would have been there. Then, maybe the regulations of the Dalkon Shield could have been different ... We now know that if you put any IUD into a woman you are going to increase the risk of pelvic inflammatory disease and, associated with that, sterility' (W. Freeland, interview, 28 July 1995).

In Canada at present, a medical device has to go through a rigorous evaluation. The manufacturer has to make an application for approval and submit documents that include the name of the product, its intended market, the purpose of the product, the form of the device, performance characteristics, specifications, the method of sterilization, how the product is made, the quality control program, full data from chemical studies and animal studies, evidence of effectiveness, clinical trial results, and indications of adverse reactions. Freeland says, 'If we haven't got that information we may have to do a clinical trial. We dialogue with the manufacturer until they have given us all of this information. If we feel the probability is OK and ... there is substantial evidence that the manufacturer's knowledge of the new device can be used for the purpose and conditions recommended by the manufacturer without undue risks to humans, and the device is effective, and the labels are OK, then we can recommend that they can market the product' (W. Freeland, interview, 28 July 1995). Those who make up the decision-making body have varying relevant educational backgrounds, such as medicine, biochemistry, engineering, and science. The members work as a team, yet answer to a hierarchy. In effect, the Canadian Medical Devices Bureau monitors the process of premarket evaluation and postmarket surveillance of the product. Ultimately, the clinical trials and identification of the various features of the product are primarily the responsibility of the manufacturer.

According to Richard Tobin, Director of the Medical Devices Bureau of the Health Protection Branch, Health Canada, regulations are fine-tuned as needed. Recent proposals address risk assessment and risk management issues of medical devices, including intrauterine devices. Product safety is the main objective of risk assessment and management. Different groups within the Canadian Medical Devices Bureau also communicate with foreign officials in similar government departments (R. Tobin, interview, 24 April 1996).

The trend today is toward global harmonization. Communication takes place annually among directors general and deputy ministers of the regulatory divisions of international medical devices bureaux. Within a group that includes officials from Canada, the United States, and Mexico, and another that includes Canada, the United States, and the United Kingdom, there are goals to explore opportunities and achieve a collaborative atmosphere among nations to ensure the safety of medical devices. Each country takes its turn to host the meeting. Similarly, officials from the U.S. FDA and the Canadian HPB meet to discuss regulations on food, drugs, and devices, as needed (R. Tobin, interview, 24 April 1996).

Tobin did not wish to comment on the rumour that industry is pressuring government to hand over more control to them. However, he did say that industry would like government to come up with global regulations, although the Medical Devices Bureau is saying it wants industry to collaborate with them. When Tobin was asked about the risk of interfering with individual and cultural values and economic systems when devising global regulations, he admitted that it can be tough to reach a consensus. He was confident, however, that there is a meeting point at which global harmonization on medical devices regulation can be achieved (R. Tobin, interview, 24 April 1996).

Madelaine Bosco and Michael McBane of the Canadian Health Coalition suggest that industry is attempting to pressure government into loosening regulations primarily because of costs. Bosco states, 'They basically don't care ... a recent information letter of proposals for regulation changes seem to indicate an attempt by the Medical Devices Bureau to harmonize with various factions, such as industry and the FDA' (M. Bosco, interview, 22 April 1996).

McBane argues that Health Canada is essentially held captive by regulatory industry. In effect, this means that industry goals are synonymous with government goals. The industry goals are to market a product and to maximize profits. 'Now, what we are faced with is significant groups of government bureaucrats who are pursuing those goals at the expense of what is good for society, what is good for the citizen, and what is good for public health' (M. McBane, interview, 24 April 1996). McBane goes on to say that the bottom line is getting the products to the market. The Canadian Health Coalition is working more closely with the Federal Minister of Health to put pressure on the Minister of Industry to strike a balance.

Director of Media Relations Karen Alcon of the Health Industry's Manufacturers Association in the United States, argues on behalf of the medical devices manufacturers on the issue of regulatory reform for medical devices: 'We are not looking to deregulate. We are basically looking for the FDA to go back to what the actual intent of the law was back in 1976 when the FDA was given the authority to regulate medical devices. What is happening is the FDA is taking an incredibly long time to approve products' (K. Alcon, interview, 25 April 1996). Alcon claims that the time-consuming FDA review process results in fewer U.S. patients getting access to breakthrough technologies, as well as U.S. companies moving their manufacturing and research and development overseas, which in turn results in job losses in the United States and less venture capital being available. Alcon states that venture capital is very important to the medical devices industry because most of the smaller companies are the true innovators of new medical technologies. Without venture capital, they can go out of business. 'What we want is the FDA to review products within the time mandated by the law which would be for ... those devices that need to prove they are substantially equivalent to those that are already on the market. They should review them in ninety days' (K. Alcon, interview, 25 April 1996). Breakthrough devices or premarket application devices, on the other hand, should be approved within 100 days. Alcon claims that at present the FDA is taking more than 700 days for such approvals.

Alcon further explains, 'Our proposals really are looking at more of a public/private partnership. We are not looking to eliminate the agency. We are not looking to reduce safety standards. We are not looking to privatize the industry. We are not looking to do any of those' (K. Alcon, interview, 25 April 1996). Instead, medical devices manufacturers want the FDA to retain its proper role as public health guardian. However, they also feel it is as important for the FDA to promote public access to medical devices as it is to prevent unsafe devices from getting on the market. The FDA's job should be solely to make sure a device is safe and effective, not to dictate other factors, such as cost-effectiveness. Alcon says: 'What we looked at is ... the European Union model. It is for approving devices. They use a third-party organization that will approve devices. We would like to use the best of the EU model system and the best of the U.S. system. What we are saying is industry would have an option. It would not be mandated' (K. Alcon, interview, 25 April 1996). In effect, she suggests that industry would have the option of going to a third party at its own cost to have a product reviewed, but the third party would have to be accredited by the FDA. Each organization would have to follow the same standards. At present, rumour has it that the FDA is in the process of fine-tuning its regulations.

The questions arise: Is a third-party option a viable alternative to the present regulatory system, or will it set up a system whereby those with the most money will get the most expedient approval of products? What is the monetary cost to the public if government and industry pontificate over who is going to get what and when? It sounds strangely like the 1970s, when questions arose about the Dalkon Shield. Billions of dollars were spent while what appeared to be obvious to most was not to others.

Central to the issue of harmful or ineffective products is the economic cost to the health-care system. For example, in British Columbia a report submitted to the Royal Commission on Health Care and Costs gives conservative estimates of the economic costs of pelvic inflammatory disease. This study covers only a small geographical terrain and a small population, but if the figures are extended to similar populations they may provide an important window to another aspect of PID. 'More than 9,000 women contract pelvic inflammatory disease each year in British Columbia (based on estimates for all of Canada for 1984–85); over 2,000 of these women become infertile as a consequence of PID. The costs to the health care system of treating these women's infections and the major consequence arising from them (ectopic pregnancy and infertility) are estimated at approximately $9 million annually in BC alone; the indirect cost to the provincial economy of lost labor productivity is approximately $5 million annually' (Canadian PID Society 1990). The estimated Canadian cost of incidence of PID, direct health-care costs, and loss of productivity during this same period is $140,158,218. A global perspective on health-care costs in relation to PID and IUD use may indeed surpass billions of dollars. Such health-care costs have an impact on the global political and social economy.

Executives of pharmaceutical companies and population control agencies must be held accountable for their role in any unethical behaviour that disregards the health of consumers. Tougher legislation must ensure that such persons serve substantial and lengthy jail terms, as well as pay monetary compensation to those injured. The responsible individuals' names should also be made public.

An in-depth analysis of the economic costs to women injured by harmful contraceptives or other reproductive technologies is needed and should be released to the public through the news media. The economic and personal costs of such injuries must be acknowledged by industry, government, population control agencies, and the Canadian and American Medical Associations. In other words, the power elite must acknowledge their role in ignoring the existence of harmful products. They must also recognize that such products disrupt family and community dynamics. Foundations or corporations that fund medical research should not have a major role in making final decisions about population control strategies.

Provincial and state health ministries must revamp their health-care guidelines for physicians. The existing processes for investigating a complaint against a physician are lengthy and do not serve the patient's interests in an efficient manner. These are often long, arduous, humiliating, and distressful processes for patients wanting closure.

Continued efforts towards global harmonization of health-care regulatory systems are a must. Tighter premarket and postsurveillance programs should continue to be developed by federal government medical agencies. Risk assessment and risk management models are a good beginning to establishing safer medical products, bearing in mind the diverse cultural and religious beliefs of various countries, especially regarding contraceptives. Leaders of such decision-making groups must also examine their biases towards people of differing economic, social, cultural, and religious backgrounds.

More stringent pre-evaluation and postsurveillance of clinical programs in underdeveloped countries should be conducted. Research groups such as UBINIG in Bangladesh should be authorized to work in conjunction with appointed government officers to monitor the method and use of any contraceptive devices being tested on people. The World Health Organization (WHO) of the United Nations should also take a greater role in monitoring clinical research programs in developing countries. However, any medical device or drug that is not approved in a developed country should not be tested in an underdeveloped country. These governments should develop and approve domestic health-care agencies that value the health of the recipients of contraceptives. Safe and realistic contraceptive methods should be available to women who want or need them, regardless of geographical location.

Dissemination of information on the safety characteristics or hazards of all contraceptives must be consistent for all people, regardless of where they live. Health-care educators in their own milieu, provided they are equipped with accurate knowledge, are most suited to providing contraceptive information to their own population.

Government should provide updated health information on potentially hazardous contraceptives through a public media vehicle such as the Internet or cable television. This information should include updated regulations and guidelines on contraceptives. Similar information could be provided through regular newspaper columns and public television. The news media must, at every opportunity, continue to investigate and report the facts about individuals or companies associated with promoting unsafe products.

Information on the administrative structure of the Dalkon Shield Claimants Trust should be made available to academics, the media, and the public upon closure of the Trust. The administrative structure should be examined for its efficiency, cost-effectiveness, and moral commitment to justice in personal injury and bankruptcy litigation. All depositories that hold documents related to the litigation surrounding the Dalkon Shield should be opened for public scrutiny. The vastness of this information could provide a manifesto of learning for scholars in the areas of law, sociology, political science, psychology, public administration, business administration, journalism, history, and public health.

In future, local advocacy groups should be established and available to victims to assist them with filing claim forms and dealing with the emotional turmoil associated with personal injury. A portion of the administrative cost could be paid to those trained to assist with paperwork and counselling of women. Some of the counselling assistance should be monitored by a representative and qualified social worker.

Charitable foundations or corporations could play a role in providing support money for such groups. Notification of location of the support centres should be sent to physicians so they can refer women to these centres. In other words, a less costly, more efficient, and more empathic web of relations should be established in larger and smaller communities for this kind of crisis. Perhaps some of these centres should be modelled after existing health collectives, such as the Vancouver Women's Health Collective and the Boston Women's Health Book Collective.

Realistic and strategic contraception education programs, along with family planning incentive programs that help provide safe medical devices as well as safe medical practices, could be implemented in underdeveloped countries. Vasectomies should be explored as an alternative contraceptive in more underdeveloped countries. In addition, education programs on contraception should be directed to men as well as women in these countries. For example, the Family Planning Association of Venezuela (PLAFAM) has an 'objective to see men fulfill their role in the nuclear family, participate in family planning, and above all, exercise their sexuality in a responsible way' ('Men also need information' 1995, 15). Domestic male health educators could also be trained to conduct seminars and clinical programs for men.

The religious and social beliefs of individual cultures must be respected when offering information and advice on all methods of contraception. Continued efforts are a must by family planning associations to 'explore and experiment with new strategies of information and communication appropriate to reach a variety of groups – the young, the illiterate and the religious' ('Working with voodoo' 1995, 3). For instance, l'Association pour la Promotion de la Famille Haitienne (PROFAMIL) works in conjunction with the highest-ranking Haitian voodoo priests to help convey family planning methods to rural populations in Haiti. Youth groups, at least in developed countries, must also continue to be part of these family planning programs.

We live in an age where new reproductive technologies, artificial joints, and heart, penile, and breast implants, among other things, are seen as progress. We assume that these commodities will add to the enjoyment of our lives. We are hopeful and remain in many respects trustful of new medical procedures and products. However, we cannot always depend on the information provided to us by pharmaceutical companies or physicians. It is imperative, therefore, that we be our own health-care keepers.

As keepers of our health, we must learn to value ourselves as intelligent human beings. We can learn to ask our doctors questions about a treatment that is supposed to help us. We must gather information from several sources and not simply take the doctor's recommendations or the pharmaceutical company's claims at face value. As consumers, we are able to effect change if we collectively object to injustice. As individuals, we can take charge of our health and refuse to let others decide what is best for us.

Epilogue: Healing

Healing for many of the female survivors of the Dalkon Shield has been long, arduous, and not always successful. The process by which these women recover has been diverse. In some cases, simply writing a letter to someone like myself has allowed women to express their anger towards the pharmaceutical company and towards some physicians and to express some of their sadness. For many, the intensity of the pain has dissipated. Some women who were left infertile have adopted children, some have remarried, and others have become stepparents. Others have continued health-care advocacy work or become teachers. Some women wrote books, others healed through the help of a sensitive therapist, and a few will heal by reading books on the Dalkon Shield story.

For others, the pain persists and eats away at them. They have not yet found room within themselves to move on. Many of these women carry guilt or regret about not having a child. Healing is a unique process that belongs to each individual. Most importantly, all of these women deserve recognition for their losses.

Those who did not incur injury from the Dalkon Shield were fortunate. One woman wrote that she had not experienced any injury from the Shield, but she empathized with those who were less fortunate. No one knows exactly why some women were not injured. We can speculate that perhaps all of the elements that needed to be in place to avoid injury were present for these women.

However, this does not deny the injuries of the victims. We cannot make the mistake of blaming hundreds of thousands of women for their injuries. The fact that over 300,000 women worldwide submitted claims for injury and 200,000 women received some kind of monetary compensation clearly confirms the scope of the tragedy. Nor can we ignore that most of the partners of these women were tragically isolated in their pain and loss. The pain these men feel for their own losses and those of the women is integral to the overall impact of the Dalkon Shield.

The children of these victims will also have to heal. It is difficult to project how these now adult children will deal with their parents' and their own suffering.

It is my hope that this book will contribute at least a little to the healing process of all those affected by the Dalkon Shield.

Segment of Interview with Michael Sheppard, Executive Director of the Dalkon Shield Claimants Trust, 14 February 1996

M.H.: Did the Trust ever take a stand on the wicking of the string of the Dalkon Shield? Was there any dispute as to whether that really was the culprit?

M.S.: The Trust has defended several cases in which plaintiffs have alleged that they developed infections as a result of 'wicking' of bacteria through the Dalkon Shield's tail string. Overall, we have been very successful in those cases and juries who have ruled in our favour have rejected that argument. In our view, the notion of 'wicking' is nothing more than 'junk science' and, in our experience, jurors have not given much money to plaintiffs making that allegation. Plaintiffs have not been successful in proving that 'wicking' caused them any harm.

M.H.: So in your view the studies that came out that said the tail string of the Dalkon Shield wicked are false.

M.S.: That expert who came out with the original study on wicking, Dr Howard Tatum, has testified for plaintiffs in cases against the Trust. He has admitted that there were serious flaws in his wicking experiments. He has also admitted that none of the women that he examined from whom the tail strings were removed ever developed infections.

M.H.: What is it then that indicates that the woman was damaged? Presumably women are getting paid because they were damaged by the Dalkon Shield?

M.S.: The medical literature most prevalent today in the United States indicates that most infections that occur with any IUD, including the Dalkon Shield, occur within thirty days of the insertion of the device. The insertion process involves the placement of the IUD through a non-sterile environment into a more sterile environment, introducing bacteria which can lead to infection. Basically, medical science now understands this to be the cause of infections associated with IUDs because most of these infections occur immediately following insertion or removal of the IUD.

M.H.: So did it have to do with the physician's ability or skill?

M.S.: Probably.

M.H.: Why did some women never have any infection from the Dalkon Shield?

M.S.: There are cases of some women who wore the Dalkon Shield for twenty-five years and never had any problems. The majority of IUDs in use twenty years ago are now off the market, and yet we still see an increasing rate of PID in women. This suggests that there is something else causing PID, and medical literature now tells us that sexually transmitted diseases are the probable cause of these infections.

M.H.: This argument has been put forth for years. Could the infection have occurred prior to the marriage?

M.S.: That's correct. It has nothing to do with the person being promiscuous; it has to do with whether they have been exposed to a sexually transmitted disease. Back in the 1970s and early 1980s when most of these cases were being tried, it was practically impossible to test for certain STDs, like chlamydia. Now, we know that chlamydia is the number one cause of PID, and it is possible today to take a blood test and find out if a woman has chlamydia or ever has had chlamydia in her whole life. This is one of the reasons the Trust is prevailing in many cases. We have asked plaintiffs to take a blood test and find out if she has ever had chlamydia. This is an alternative cause of PID. Most of the experts today will tell you that sexually transmitted diseases, not IUDs, cause infections. Advances in the medicine over the last twenty years are the reason why the Trust has been so successful in litigation. It has nothing to do with promiscuity or the morals of the person. We just know more now than was known twenty years ago.

M.H: So why are women still being awarded settlements based on claims that they were injured from the use of the Dalkon Shield, marketed and distributed by Robins, if in fact they were injured because of the lack of skill of a physician? Is this evidence based on an article published by Dr Stephen Mumford?

M.S.: People often sue even when it is not 'legitimate,' i.e., even though there may be no grounds for legal liability. The Tatum study and the litigation fever that stemmed from it and surrounded the Dalkon Shield in the late 1970s and early 1980s generated thousands of suits at a time when the medical knowledge of insertion risks and STDs was not what it is now. This forced Robins into bankruptcy to centralize all claims to be handled through one claims facility. The terms of the consensus plan eventually developed by all parties and approved by the court and claimants was designed to end all litigation and encourage the resolution of claims by settlement, rather than adversarial [means]. Thus, the plan and the CRF [Claimants Resolution Facility] contained certain presumptions of eligibility for compensation for the categories of injuries normally claimed by Dalkon Shield users or their family members, tilting the files in favour of the claimants during these voluntary settlement steps of the CRF process, and evaluation criteria of Option 3. In the latter alternative causes of infection are considered and do affect claim value. Medical actions or omissions do not. This permits claims to be finished more efficiently without the delay and expense associated with the adversarial proceedings and legal technicalities. This has worked quite well. The Trust has resolved 98 per cent of the claims before it. Over 85 per cent of the finished claims were concluded by settlement. Indeed, 98 per cent of claims receiving offers from the Trust of over $6,000 accepted those offers. All claimants who were paid more than $725 originally are receiving pro rata payments of excess funds that the Trust hopes will amount to 90 per cent of their original awards. But when a claimant rejects her offers and chooses to seek greater recoveries through the adversarial system, the plan and the Claimants Resolution Facility (CRF) are clear that the Trust can and must use the defences available to it that may very well defeat the claim entirely. Your mention of Dr Mumford must be a reference to the article 'Was the Dalkon Shield a Safe and Effective Intrauterine Device?' [*Fertility and Sterility*, 6 June 1992]. That article is consistent with the Trust's view of this issue.

M.H.: Is Dr Tatum now liable for his apparently unfounded accusations about the tail string of the Dalkon Shield? Where does this place Dr Tatum's credibility in the scientific research world?

M.S.: I have no opinion on these two issues. Neither is relevant to the successful operation of the Trust.

M.H.: Does this change the Dalkon Shield story markedly? Was there a mistake in blaming Robins for marketing an IUD that was alleged to have caused harm to women?

M.S.: Whether this changes the 'Dalkon Shield story' depends upon whose story you are referencing. The version still promoted by the plaintiffs' lawyers is that the Dalkon Shield was unreasonably dangerous. The Trust's view is that the medical research does not support that version in general, and that the medical evidence does not in particular cases prove that the Dalkon Shield was the source of alleged injuries. It is not fruitful in hindsight to label either filing suits against Robins or Robins' entry into bankruptcy as a 'mistake.' The reality is that, given our tort system and the rampant litigation in this country relating to all types of products, Robins was forced into bankruptcy to resolve this problem. Once it became a huge problem, the right thing to do was to finish the litigation relating to the device and develop a method of processing claims that reduced, as much as possible, the transaction costs associated with tort claims resolution. The plan and the CRF were designed to do that. The Trust's experience to date has proved them successful.

Segment of Interview with Miles Lord, Lawyer and Former Judge Who Presided Over the Charges against Robins, 15 April 1996

M.H.: The Dalkon Shield Trust is stating that the original theory about the wicking of the tail string of the Dalkon Shield is now considered 'junk science.' What is your opinion about this suggestion?

M.L.: If that is 'junk science' then a lantern will not burn. What I mean is that the wicking is such a simple principle. The theory of fluid rising in a capillary is so simple. According to that [junk science label] we were in the dark until the light bulb came because you couldn't wick anything.

M.H.: Presently, the Dalkon Shield Claimants Trust is suggesting that the doctors' inexperience in terms of inserting the actual IUD was the prime problem. What is your opinion about this statement?

M.L.: They started by joining the doctors as defendants and then they stopped. After all of the statutes of limitations have run out they are then free to blame the doctor because nobody can do anything about it.

M.H.: Do you think it is political?

M.L.: It is economic politics, of course. It is totally political. It's corporate conduct at its worst. Now [pharmaceutical companies] are spending billions of dollars to advertise about their research. The truth is they do almost no research. They wait for some little company to discover something and then they go and buy the company. For example, Minnesota (where I am from) is full of small companies where inventions have been made and taken over by the big pharmaceutical companies. I should have put some of the Robins' defence attorneys in jail for the things they did, some of which were done in my courtroom, but it moved so fast and they were so clever. They escaped punishment.

Gerry's Story (letter to Gerry's lawyer)

April 24, 1990

Dear Bob:

When Irene and I met with you earlier this month you told me that you felt it important that I finally come to terms with the results of Irene's use of the Dalkon Shield. Irene has told me this for years and I know you are both right. There is nothing in this world I would like more to do, but the time is not yet right. As long as there is any possibility that Irene might need me for emotional support I must be ready. I am very much afraid that when I finally allow myself to talk to someone about those events I will break ...

The hardest thing I have ever done in my life and the event I relive almost every day of my life was to walk up to Irene's bedside after the septic abortion and to try to be strong for her, to comfort and reassure her when I myself was devastated. I don't remember how I came to be in the hallway outside her room at the time of the abortion. How I hate that word. I may have been visiting her and been sent out. I may have been on my way to the room, I don't know. I stood outside the door, listening to the nurse coaching Irene and talking to her. Irene was in pain, she was delirious, she was crying. She was totally out of control emotionally. The nurse left the room and walked past me. She was carrying a white enamel tray covered by a white towel with an edge sewn in yellow thread. I shall never forget it. It carried my dead baby. I had to be strong for Irene. I tried to comfort and reassure her that the nightmare was over and that she would be fine now, we would have another baby. She changed back and forth from being delirious, to crying uncontrollably, to apologizing for losing our baby. I stayed strong, I was sent home and the nurse took care of Irene. I went to tell my parents it was over and I went home to my other kids. I had to be strong for them. My body ached all over from tension. My chest burned ... my mind was racing with emotions of hate, depression, rage and sorrow. I buried myself in the tasks at hand ...

For years Irene and I went from Doctor to Doctor to try to understand the pain that resulted from the abortion. We were told many different things, including that it was all in her head. I remember visiting her in hospital and she was crying because no one believed her. They said it was emotional. I must admit that I sometimes suspected this was the case, but tried to support her. Those were extremely stressful years for us. We didn't know if she would ever be free of pain. Nobody was ever willing or competent enough to tie the pain to the Dalkon Shield infection and PID. Only when the Dalkon Shield scandal became public did the Doctors guardedly admit to the cause. Our own Doctor quit and left Canada about the time the truth about Dalkon Shield was filtering out. All Irene's records were destroyed. Possibly he was afraid of litigation.

One day while driving down the road with my son John he began to talk about the baby we had lost. Irene has talked to both of our kids about those events. I cannot talk about it at all so I had never discussed it much with either of them. John mentioned that the baby had been a boy. He might as well have driven a spike into my heart. I had never wanted to know if it was a girl or a boy. I guess it was easier to deal with it ... I don't know why, but it is now harder for me to handle than ever before. I often wonder what my other son would have been like ...

Sincerely,
Gerry

Glossary

The following terms are commonly used in describing the Dalkon Shield litigation process.

Alternative Dispute Resolution (ADR) An appeal process whereby a lawyer representing the claimant and a lawyer representing the Dalkon Shield Trust meet to negotiate a higher settlement for the claimant, and the claimant has an opportunity to argue her or his case. A referee mediates the discussion and then decides on a settlement based on the arguments presented by both sides.

Arbitration The hearing and determination of a dispute by an impartial referee selected or agreed upon by the parties concerned. The claimants opted for this process only after they rejected a settlement offered from Option 3 process.

Breland case In April 1986, a class action lawsuit filed against Aetna insurance company, A.H. Robins's insurer, by persons claiming Dalkon Shield injuries. The lawsuit, *Breland vs. The Aetna Casualty and Surety Company* was pending in the Eastern District of Virginia, where the Robins petition for reorganization of its assets under Chapter 11 was pending. In the Breland case, the plaintiffs asserted numerous claims against Aetna and attacked the settlement agreement. As part of the Robins reorganization plan, Robins and Aetna settled the controversies between themselves.

Chapter 7 A bankruptcy code whereby a company loses all of its assets.

Chapter 11 A bankruptcy code whereby a company is allowed to reorganize its assets and come up with a plan to pay its debt. The A.H. Robins Company reorganized itself by merging with American Home Products Corporation. In essence, Robins filed for bankruptcy, but also retained $750 million worth of AHP shares, which were given to Robins's shareholders.

Contingency fee A lawyer's fee that is similar to a commission. The lawyer does not receive a fee for his or her services until the client has been awarded monetary compensation from a lawsuit. If the client does not receive any award, the lawyer does not receive a contingency fee.

Dalkon Shield Claimants Trust An organizational body established to hold funds for persons filing claims for compensation for personal injury caused by the Dalkon Shield.

Option 1 A category of personal injury claim established by the Dalkon Shield Claimants Trust. This category covers claimants with minimal injuries and women who cannot prove injury because of missing medical records. Settlements for these claims are between $100 and $750.

Option 2 A category of personal injury claim established by the Dalkon Shield Claimants Trust. This category covers women who have medical records proving they have used a Shield.

Option 3 A category of personal injury claim established by the Dalkon Shield Claimants Trust. This category covers women who have medical records that can be used to prove their injuries were incurred from using the Dalkon Shield and no other IUD. If a settlement offer is not acceptable to the claimant, she can counter the offer.

Option 4 A category of personal injury claim established by the Dalkon Shield Claimants Trust. This category makes it possible for claimants to file claims for injuries that might occur in the future as a result of the Dalkon Shield.

Pro rata distribution A distribution of excess funds to claimants based on their original monetary settlement from the Dalkon Shield Trust Fund. Claimants received three additional payments from excess funds, which together amounted to 100 per cent of the original award given to a claimant. For example, if a claimant received $50,000 initially, she or he then received another $50,000 in pro rata distribution of funds.

Reorganization plan A plan designed to reorganize Robins's assets once the company received approval to file for Chapter 11 bankruptcy. The reorganization plan allowed money to be placed in the Dalkon Shield Trust Fund to pay claimants.

Settlement conference A negotiation process available to claimants and their lawyers who were dissatisfied with their original award above $20,000. It was an opportunity to negotiate before going to trial.

Sixth Amended and Restated Disclosure Statement The sixth version of the A.H. Robins reorganization plan; the relevant facts and figures were compiled into this report.

Litigation Chronology

This information is derived from accurate published calendars of events.

1972: The Dalkon Shield lawsuit is filed in Michigan.

2 August 1985: Four Minnesota attorneys representing nearly 2,000 claimants – John Cochrane of St Paul, Minnesota, and Joseph S. Friedberg, Ronald I. Meshbesher, and James Hovland, of Minneapolis – file a class action suit on behalf of all Dalkon Shield claimants. A.H. Robins files its bankruptcy petition the same month.

22 August 1985: The Minnesota attorneys refile their request for a class action within the context of the bankruptcy proceeding. Judge Merhige puts the request on hold pending Robins's reorganization.

9 November 1985: Judge Merhige grants Robins's motion that all Dalkon Shield cases filed in the United States be transferred to Richmond, Virginia. Subsequently, the U.S. Court of Appeal for the Fourth Circuit upholds the transfer order with some procedural modifications.

26 November 1985: Robins requests an extension to its original 31 December 1985 deadline for filing its reorganization plan. A new deadline is set for 31 March 1986.

27 December 1985: Robins unsuccessfully requests the court to im-

pound the list of Dalkon Shield claimants, maintaining that the plaintiffs' counsel would solicit clients.

8 January 1986: The federal bankruptcy trustee for the case, William C. White, appoints a three-person equity security holders committee.

4 March 1986: Judge Merhige grants the bankruptcy trustee's motion to dissolve the plaintiffs' thirty-eight-member committee after it seeks to replace its special counsel, Murray Drabkin of Washington, DC. The committee views Drabkin as insufficiently aggressive in challenging the bankruptcy system as it addresses mass tort cases. Judge Merhige agrees with the trustee that the committee is not functioning as it should. Drabkin stays on in his post with the understanding that the judge will appoint a new committee. On the same day ten attorneys representing eighty Dalkon Shield claimants ask Judge Merhige to disqualify himself from the case. Merhige refuses.

12 March 1986: The assistant U.S. attorney asks the court to appoint an independent trustee to take over Robins's operation, alleging postbankruptcy payments of fees to contractors and deferred compensation to Robins executives totalling $750 million.

19 March 1986: The federal bankruptcy trustee names a new five-member committee of claimants to represent the plaintiffs.

21 March 86: Robins announces that it had dismissed its outside bankruptcy counsel, the San Francisco firm of Murphy, Weir and Butler. The company gives no public explanation for the sudden dismissal, and in early April it retains the firm of Skadden, Arps, Slate, Meagher and Flom of New York. One rumour suggests that Robins blames Murphy, Weir and Butler for the improper payments to contractors and Robins executives, but a contradictory report states that Robins executives made the payment decisions.

On the same day, Robins announces the early retirement of its in-house general counsel, William A. Forrest, Jr, who had been with the company for twenty years. Forrest says he is retiring for personal reasons.

On the same day, the committee of equity security holders requests an extension of the 31 March deadline by which Robins is to propose its reorganization plan. A few days later Robins also requests an extension. Judge Merhige sets a new deadline of 30 June, which could be extended again.

28 March 1986: Merhige demands that Robins retrieve $1.7 million in improper payments to Robins executives, plus interest. By May, the company has arranged for most of the money to be repaid.

April 1986: An application to extend the deadline to file claims is filed by the Vancouver and Winnipeg Health Collectives. Judge Merhige allows that any claim postmarked by midnight of 30 April 1986 will be accepted. This allows an additional 19,000 claims worldwide.

April 1986: The Breland class action is filed against Aetna Life and Casualty Company.

April 1987: After being granted five extensions, Robins files a proposed reorganization plan.

June 1987: A $15 million fund is established to pay for reconstructive surgery and *in vitro* fertilization for women under the age of forty. The maximum payment to each individual is $15,000 and will be deducted from the woman's final settlement.

July 1987: Robins's stockholders appeal the establishment of the fund for reconstructive surgery and *in vitro* fertilization, arguing that the fund is premature. The appeal is upheld.

November 1987: Robins values claims at $812 million to $1.22 billion. The official claimants committee values claims at $4.2 billion to $7 billion.

December 1987: Judge Merhige rules that the total value of Dalkon Shield claims is $2.375 billion.

January 1988: Robins's Board of Directors accepts the offer from American Home Products to buy the Robins company for $3.27 billion. Of this amount, $2.375 billion is placed in a trust to pay Dalkon Shield claimants. $750 million worth of AHP shares are paid to Robins's stockholders, contrary to existing bankruptcy law. The law states that creditors (including claimants) must be paid first.

February 1988: Clairborne Robins, Sr, and Clairborne Robins, Jr, add $10 million to the trust fund in return for immunity from future liability. This raises the amount of the fund to $2.475 billion.

April 1988: The *Sixth Amended and Restated Disclosure Statement*, which describes the Robins reorganization plan, and accompanying ballot is mailed to claimants or their attorney. The *Statement* includes seven covering letters, including one from the official claimants committee, which all say that the plan should be accepted. Judge Merhige does not allow dissenting views to be included. Many claimants never see the plan, as their vote is cast by proxy by their attorney.

May 1988: A coalition of claimants' groups is formed in Washington, DC. It is unanimously decided that the *Sixth Amended and Restated Disclosure Statement* must be rejected because it is unfair, inadequate, and contrary to existing law.

June 1988: The precedent-setting mandatory class action suit against Aetna Life and Casualty Company is upheld by Judge Merhige. This allows Aetna to limit its liability for the Dalkon Shield even though the company is not in bankruptcy and it participated in the cover-up of the hazards of the Dalkon Shield.

July 1988: The *Sixth Amended and Restated Disclosure Statement* (the plan) is accepted by the claimants. Judge Merhige confirms the plan even though it changes existing Chapter 11 bankruptcy law.

August 1988: Public Citizen Advocacy, an American consumer organization, appeals the *Sixth Amended and Restated Disclosure Statement*.

1989–95: Under the terms of the reorganization plan, claimants receive initial compensation for injuries.

December 1995: The first pro rata distribution payments are sent to claimants: 60 per cent of the claimants' original settlement is paid.

November 1996: Pro rata distribution of funds is issued to claimants. Claimants receive 25 per cent of their original settlement. Lawyers are able to take a limit of 10 per cent off the top of the pro rata distribution.

1999: Final pro rata distribution of between 5 and 15 per cent is expected at the end of 1999.

Number of Official Claims by Region as of 5 February 1987

The Americas (not U.S. and Canada)		Southwest Asia and Africa		Europe		East Asia	
Argentina	43	Botswana	3	Austria	8	Australia	5049
Bahamas	11	Cameroon	1	Belgium	39	Bangladesh	52
Belize	2	Egypt	3	Denmark	85	India	55
Brazil	1135	Ethiopia	3	W. Germany	260	Japan	8
Chile	2	Iran	4	Finland	79	Malaysia	9
Colombia	18	Israel	236	France	105	New Zealand	474
Costa Rica	56	Kenya	32	Greece	17	Pakistan	6
Dominican		Kuwait	1	Iceland	1	Papua New	
Republic	5	Lesotho	4	Ireland	349	Guinea	8
Ecuador	6	Liberia	2	Italy	27	Philippines	508
El Salvador	31	Malawi	2	Luxembourg	2	Singapore	1
Grenada	1	Nigeria	30	Malta	2	Sri Lanka	14
Guatemala	15	Oman	1	Netherlands	1473	Taiwan	696
Honduras	2	Saudi Arabia	10	Norway	254	Thailand	3
Jamaica	15	South Africa	283	Poland	2	Vanuatu	1
Mexico	15	Swaziland	2	Portugal	3	Vietnam	1
Nicaragua	6	Syria	2	Spain	11	W. Samoa	1
Panama	13	Tanzania	3	Sweden	479	**Total**	**6886**
Paraguay	2	Tonga	2	Switzerland	6		
Peru	1	Tunisia	2	UK	3494		
Trinidad	2	Turkey	28	Yugoslavia	1		
Venezuela	1	Uganda	2	**Total**	**6697**		
Total	**1382**	U.A.E.	4				
		Zaire	1				
		Zimbabwe	19				
		Total	**680**				

All original claims from the following countries did not comply with Bankruptcy Court protocol and were thereby summarily denied: Algeria, Antigua,

Barbados, Central African Republic, Gambia, Ghana, Haiti, Indonesia, South Korea, St. Vincent, Sudan. The total number of international claims as of 5 February 1987 (including Canada, with 3,027 claims) was 18,689. The total number of U.S. claims as of 2 February 1987 was 161,351.

Data source: U.S. Bankruptcy Court, Richmond, Virginia. No known update is available.

The U.S. monetary compensation for each Bangladeshi woman and man who filed a claim was from $3,675.91 U.S. for six women; $2,606.56 for six women (one woman died and her husband collected on her behalf); $835.43 for nine women; $668.35 for one woman, $568.10 for two women; $484.56 for twenty-three women (two women died and their husbands received monetary compensation on their behalf); and $200.50 for sixteen men (Akhter 1995, 131–33).

References

Akhter, F. 1995. *Resisting Norplant: Women's Struggle in Bangladesh against Coercion and Violence*. Dhaka, Bangladesh: Narigrantha Prabartana.

Anselmi, Kathy Kaby. 1994. 'Women's response to reproductive trauma secondary to contraceptive iatrogenesis: A phenomenological approach to the Dalkon Shield.' PhD diss., University of Pennsylvania, UM1 Dissertation Services.

Arocha, Z. 1983. 'Miamian gets 4.9 million in suit over contraceptive.' *Miami News*, 15 December, cover page.

Associated Press. 1988. 'Merger completed as Dalkon fund set up.' *Vancouver Sun*, 17 March, A10.

Borditsky, R., Fisher, W., Sand, M. 1995. 'The Canadian Contraception Study.' *SOGC* (July): 22–25.

Boston Women's Health Book Collective. 1992. *The New Our Bodies, Ourselves*. New York: Simon & Schuster.

Buchan, H.,Villard-Mackintosh, L., Vessey, M., Yeates, D., McPherson, K. 1990. 'Epidemiology of pelvic inflammatory disease in parous women with special reference to intrauterine device use.' *British Journal of Obstetrics and Gynaecology* 97: 780–88.

Canadian Broadcasting Corporation. 1996. 'The Human Laboratory.' *Witness*. 23 January [Television program]. Purchased from British Broadcasting Corporation (BBC), *Horizon* program, original title: 'Every woman's dream.'

Canadian Pelvic Inflammatory Disease (PID) Society. 1990. 'Submission to the Royal Commission on Health Care and Costs.' 10 October.

Canadian Press. 1988. 'Dalkon settlement offer draws fire.' *The Ottawa Citizen*, 10 December, A20.

– 1987. 'Bankruptcy hearing "major step" for women seeking compensation in Dalkon Shield case.' *The Ottawa Citizen*, 23 July, D6.

Christian, C.D. 1974. 'Maternal death associated with an intrauterine device.' *American Journal Obstetrics Gynecology* 119.4 (May–August): 441–44.

Courie, E. 1986. 'The A.H. Saga.' *ABA Journal* (1 July): 57–58.

Cramer, D., et al. 1985. 'Tubal infertility and the intrauterine device.' 312.15: 941–47.

Daling, J.R., et al. 1985. 'Primary tubal infertility in relation to use of an intrauterine device.' *New England Journal of Medicine* 312.15: 937–41.

'Dalkon: A contraceptive "holocaust," American justice in question: Women fighting for inquiry into Dalkon Shield horror.' 1988. *Calgary Herald*, 7 August, B5.

Davis, H. 1972. 'Intrauterine contraceptive devices: Present status and future prospects.' *American Journal Obstetrics Gynecology* 114.1 (1 September): 134–51.

– 1970. 'The shield intrauterine device.' *American Journal Obstetrics Gynecology* (1 February): 455–56.

Egan, A. 1988. 'The damage done: The endless saga of the Dalkon Shield.' *Village Voice* (5 July): 23–30.

Eschenbach, D.A. 1992. 'Earth, motherhood, and the intrauterine device.' *Fertility and Sterility* 57.6:1177–79.

'Ethics for scientific researchers.' 1971. *Canadian Medical Association Journal* 105 (7 August): 137–38.

FDA. 1996. Correspondence from M.T. Rivero, information technician, 29 January.

Fido, M., and Fido, K. 1996. *The World's Worst Medical Mistakes*. Great Britain: Sevenoaks Books.

Franklin, R.R., and Brockman, D.K. 1990. *In Pursuit of Fertility: A Consultation with a Specialist*. New York: Henry Holt and Company.

The Gazette, Montreal. 1993. 'Doctors urged to back compensation claims by Dalkon victims.' *The Ottawa Citizen*. 8 September, A12.

Gladwell, M. 1989. 'Lawyers' fees in Dalkon Shield case under fire.' *Washington Post*, 22 January, H8–H9.

Global Television Network. 1996. 'Hour of Power.' 12 May. [Television program].

Grant, N. 1992. *Selling of Contraception*. Columbus, OH: Ohio State University Press.

Grimes, D.A. 1987. 'Intrauterine devices and pelvic inflammatory disease.' *Contraception* 36.1: 97–109.

Health Protection Branch, Health and Welfare Canada. 1974. 'Suspension of the Dalkon Shield Intrauterine Devices.' News release, 28 June.

Hicks, K. 1994. *Surviving the Dalkon Shield IUD: Women v. the Pharmaceutical Industry.* New York: Teachers College Press, Columbia University.

Kirkey, S. 1996. 'Doctors get poor marks for courtesy: Patients fight back with hundreds of complaints.' *The Ottawa Citizen,* 17 February, A1–A2.

Laforet, Megan, Producer. 1994. *Infertility: To Have a Child* [Video]. Dreams and Realities Production in association with Infertility Awareness Association of Canada.

Marshall, B.R., Hepler, J.K., Scott R.H., Zirbel, C.C. 1974. 'The Dalkon Shield in nulliparous women.' *American Journal Obstetrics Gynecology* 118.2: 186–89.

McKay, A. 1996. 'Rural parents' attitudes toward school-based sexual health education.' *The Canadian Journal of Human Sexuality* 5.1 (Spring): 15.

'Men also need information.' 1995. *Forum* 11.2 (December): 15.

Merrill, K., Burd, L.I., and VerBurg, D.J. 1974. 'Laparoscopic removal of intraperitoneal Dalkon Shields: A report of three cases.' *American Journal Obstetrics Gynecology* 118.8 (15 April): 1146–48.

Mintz, M. 1989. 'When expediency, not law, prevails.' *Legal Times* (11 September): 28–33.

– 1985. *At Any Cost: Corporate Greed, Women, and the Dalkon Shield.* New York: Pantheon Books.

Mishell, D.R., Jr. 1985. 'Current status of intrauterine devices.' *The New England Journal* 312.15: 984–85.

Morris, T. 1988. 'Claimants approve Robins plan.' *Richmond Times-Dispatch,* 19 July, A-1.

Mumford, S., & Kessel, E. 1992. 'Was the Dalkon Shield a safe and effective intrauterine device? The conflict between case-control and clinical trial study findings.' *Fertility and Sterility* 57.6 (6 June): 1151–73.

NBC. 1995. 'Breast implants.' *Dateline.* 10 October. [Television program].

'On the needless hounding of a safe contraceptive.' 1995. *The Economist* (2 September): 75–76.

Ostergard, D.R. 1973. 'Intrauterine contraception in nulliparas with the Dalkon Shield.' *American Journal Obstetrics Gynecology* 116.8: 1088–91.

Owen, F.B. 1980. Letter to doctors, 19 December.

Paavonen, J. 1995. 'Chlamydia, gonorrhea, and reproductive health.' *Journal SOGC*, 1067–75.

Parsons, A.H., Parsons, P.B.N. 1995. *Hippocrates Now! Is Your Doctor Ethical?* Toronto: University of Toronto Press.

Perry, S., and Dawson, J. (1985). *Nightmare: Women and the Dalkon Shield.* New York: Macmillan.

Polon, A.J. 1973. 'Destruction of the Dalkon Shield literature.' Memo to Bob Hogsett, et al. 31 October.

Rioux, J.E. 1993. 'The intrauterine device today.' *Journal SOGC* 15: 921–24.

– 1986. 'Long-term study of the safety of the Dalkon Shield and Gyn-T 200 intrauterine devices.' *Canadian Medical Association Journal* 134: 747–51.

Scully, D. 1980. *Men Who Control Women's Health: The Miseducation of Obstetricians-Gynecologists.* Boston: Houghton-Mifflin.

Seaman, B. 1969 [rev. 1995]. *The Doctors' Case against the Pill.* New York: Hunter House.

Snowden, R., and Pearson, B. 1984. 'Pelvic infection: A comparison of the Dalkon Shield and three other intrauterine devices.' *British Medical Journal* 288: 1570–73.

Sobol, R.B. 1991. *Bending the Law: The Story of the Dalkon Shield Bankruptcy.* Chicago: University of Chicago Press.

Stewart, W. 1995. *Belly Up: The Spoils of Bankruptcy.* Toronto: McClelland and Stewart.

Tatum, H.J. 1977. 'Clinical aspects of intrauterine contraception: circumspection.' *Fertility and Sterility* 28.1: 3–28.

– 1976. 'Transport of bacteria by the Dalkon Shield.' *JAMA* 235.7 (16 February): 704–5.

– 1975a. 'The Dalkon Shield controversy: Structural and bacteriological studies of IUD tails.' *JAMA* 231.7 (17 February): 711–17.

– 1975b. 'Metallic copper as an intrauterine contraceptive agent.' *American Journal Obstetrics Gynecology* 117.5: 602–18.

– 1975c. 'Morphological studies of Dalkon Shield tails removed from patients.' *Contraception* 11.4: 465–77.

Tatum, H.J., and Connell, E.B. 1986. 'A decade of intrauterine contraception: 1976 to 1986.' *Fertility and Sterility* 46.2: 173–92.

United States Bankruptcy Court Eastern District of Virginia, Richmond Division. 1988. *Sixth Amended and Restated Disclosure Statement Pursuant to Section 1125 of the Bankruptcy Code* (The Plan). 28 March.

United States Department of Health, Education, and Welfare, Food and Drug Administration. 1978. 'Second report on intrauterine contraceptive devices.' Washington, DC: Government Printing Office, December.

Vessey, M.P., Lawless, M., McPherson, K., Yeates, D. 1983. 'Fertility after stopping the use of intrauterine contraceptive device.' *British Medical Journal* 286 (8 January): 106.

Vessey, M.P., Yeates D., Flavel, R., McPherson, K. 1981. 'Pelvic inflammatory disease and the intrauterine device: Findings in a large cohort study.' *British Medical Journal* 282: 855–59.

Washington, A.E., et al. 1991. 'Assessing risk for pelvic infammatory disease and its sequelae.' *JAMA* 266: 18.

Weld, M. 1996. 'Female education: The solution to the population crisis.' *Humanist in Canada* (June): 32.

'Working with voodoo.' *Forum* 11.2 (December): 3.

Index

[redacted]

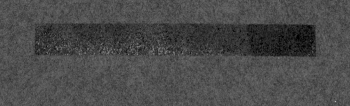